Alternative Therapies FOR Epilepsy

Orrin Devinsky, MD
Director, NYU Epilepsy Center
Professor of Neurology, Neurosurgery & Psychiatry
New York University Langone School of Medicine
New York, New York

Steven C. Schachter, MD
Professor of Neurology
Harvard Medical School
Chief Academic Officer
Center for Integration of Medicine and Innovative Technology
Boston, Massachusetts

Steven V. Pacia, MD
Associate Professor of Neurology
New York University Langone School of Medicine
Director, Division of Neurology and the Epilepsy Center
Lenox Hill Hospital
New York, New York

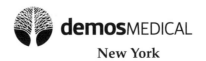
demosMEDICAL
New York

Visit our website at www.demosmedpub.com

ISBN: 978-1-9362-8732-1
e-book ISBN: 978-1-6170-5066-4

Acquisitions Editor: Beth Barry
Compositor: The Manila Typesetting Company

Medicine is an ever-changing science. Research and clinical experience are continually expanding our knowledge, in particular our understanding of proper treatment and drug therapy. The authors, editors, and publisher have made every effort to ensure that all information in this book is in accordance with the state of knowledge at the time of production of the book. Nevertheless, the authors, editors, and publisher are not responsible for errors or omissions or for any consequences from application of the information in this book and make no warranty, express or implied, with respect to the contents of the publication. Every reader should examine carefully the package inserts accompanying each drug and should carefully check whether the dosage schedules mentioned therein or the contraindications stated by the manufacturer differ from the statements made in this book. Such examination is particularly important with drugs that are either rarely used or have been newly released on the market.

Library of Congress Cataloging-in-Publication Data

Devinsky, Orrin.
  Alternative therapies for epilepsy / Orrin Devinsky, Steven C. Schachter, Steven V. Pacia.
    p. ; cm.
  Includes bibliographical references and index.
  ISBN 978-1-936287-32-1—ISBN 978-1-61705-066-4 (e-book)
  I. Schachter, Steven C. II. Pacia, Steven, 1962- III. Title.
  [DNLM: 1. Epilepsy—therapy. 2. Complementary Therapies. WL 385]

  616.85'3—dc23

                                    2012014977

Special discounts on bulk quantities of Demos Medical Publishing books are available to corporations, professional associations, pharmaceutical companies, health care organizations, and other qualifying groups. For details, please contact:
Special Sales Department
Demos Medical Publishing, LLC
11 West 42nd Street, 15th Floor
New York, NY 10036
Phone: 800-532-8663 or 212-683-0072
Fax: 212-941-7842
E-mail: rsantana@demosmedpub.com

Printed in the United States of America by Hamilton Printing

12 13 14 15 / 5 4 3 2 1

Contents

Preface

For 1 in 3 people with epilepsy (PWE), seizures are incompletely controlled by antiepileptic drugs (AEDs). While highly effective and safe for selected PWEs with drug-resistant seizures, brain surgery is either unavailable or not an option for many others. Newer AEDs may offer a better adverse-events profile compared with the older AEDs, but many have side effects that impair quality of life in a significant proportion of PWEs. These effects include decreased cognitive abilities and psychiatric complications, even when seizures are well controlled.

Against this background of incomplete seizure control and debilitating side effects of therapy, PWE often turn to alternative treatments, otherwise known as complementary and alternative medicine (CAM). Defined by the National Center for Complementary and Alternative Medicine as a group of diverse medical and health care systems, practices, and products that are not generally considered part of conventional medicine as practiced in the West (e.g., the United States), CAM comprises 4 general domains of practice: mind-body medicine (meditation, prayer, mental healing, art, music, dance); biologically based practices (use of substances found in nature such as herbs, foods, vitamins, animal compounds); manipulative and body-based practices (chiropractic or osteopathic manipulation, massage); and energy medicine (biofield and bioelectromagnetic therapies). In addition to these specific modalities, CAM may be embodied in medical systems, such as homeopathy, naturopathy, Ayurveda, and traditional Chinese medicine, each of which is characterized by a complex and unique system of diagnostics and therapeutics.

Surveys indicate that up to 1 in 2 PWE has tried an alternative therapy. Physicians need to be sufficiently knowledgeable to inform and advise their patients about the potential risks and benefits associated with these therapies. This book summarizes for treating physicians published data on the efficacy and risks of many alternative therapies. As academic epileptologists, our approach is to objectively present the available evidence in the context of the Western allopathic tradition so that physicians similarly trained in biologically based therapies can apply this information to the care of their patients, and so that patients and families with epilepsy can benefit from what we have been able to learn from the published literature about CAM therapies for epilepsy.

Physicians make decisions based on evidence from high-quality, published clinical studies. Unfortunately, the evidence base supporting the use or avoidance of CAM modalities for PWE is largely nonexistent or inadequate at present. However, this is a fast-moving field, and enhanced study designs will likely help clarify which therapies should or should not be used for patients with particular seizure types, AED side effects, or epilepsy-related comorbidities.

The doctor-patient relationship still remains the most important component in the practice of medicine. We hope that this volume helps to strengthen this relationship, stimulates new research, and fosters a broader perspective of health for people with epilepsy.

The authors thank Tracy Ma for her editorial assistance.

1

Alternative Therapies in Epilepsy: An Overview

When a scientist doesn't know the answer to a problem, he is ignorant. When he has a hunch as to what the result is, he is uncertain. And when he is pretty damn sure of what the result is going to be, he is still in some doubt.

Richard Feynman (1)

The relationships and roles of mainstream medicine (MM) and complementary and alternative medicine (CAM) continue to evolve. For people with epilepsy, MM offers medications, dietary therapies, surgery, and vagus nerve stimulation. These therapies are supported by science's gold standard: the double-blind, placebo-controlled randomized trial (DB-PC-RT). Yet most patients cared for by MM still experience seizures, side effects, or both (2). Medication side effects are underappreciated by physicians (3). People with treatment-resistant epilepsy financially burden the health care system (4). They often undergo extensive testing, require emergency room or inpatient care, and may be treated by surgical removal of epileptic brain tissue. These are the patients who often use CAM therapies. The gap between what MM offers and what patients need is enormous. Complementary and alternative medicine helps to fill this gap, but how well? This book explores the evidence on CAM in epilepsy care.

Science-based medical care and prevention is a recent invention. The first epilepsy therapy with proven efficacy was potassium bromide in 1857. The next year, Sieveking (5) wrote that "there is not a substance in the material medica, there is scarcely a substance in the world, capable of passing through the gullet of man, that has not at one time or other enjoyed a reputation of being an anti-epileptic" (p. 256). Sieveking recorded a spectrum of "alternative therapies," including tourniquets on a seizing extremity, diets, rest, and herbal baths. Yet his mainstream therapies (e.g., bleeding) are now alternative or abandoned. The distinction between MM and CAM is fluid over time and space.

Mainstream medicine and CAM can form a continuum of care. The Navajo often receive complementary health care from the Indian Health Service and native healers. They go to the native healers for common disorders such as arthritis, depression, and diabetes, as well as "bad luck" (6). One observer commented, "Physicians and other healers simply remove obstacles to the body's restoration of homeostasis, or, as the Navajo say, to harmony. . . . An alternative model [of healing] might include emotional, social, or spiritual phenomena equally as significant to healing as are biochemical phenomena" (7). We all recognize the tremendous value of offering kindness, caring, hope, and information for individuals with physical and emotional problems. These form an essential element of both MM and CAM approaches to health but are often better articulated in CAM. Indeed, in towns like Roseto, PA, where heart attack and stroke rates are remarkably low given genetics, diet, smoking, and other known risk factors, only the depth of community connections can explain their remarkable health (8). Similarly, in Dharamsala, Tibet, many people see both Western physicians and traditional healers. The CAM practitioners use plants and acupuncture and view an individual's terrain like a garden's soil (9). For acute disorders like appendicitis or a broken bone, one goes to Western doctors. For chronic problems that take time to treat, one goes to an Eastern healer (9). This parallels the approach by many Navajo. It is a concept that deserves careful study. Rates of disability due to chronic pain and depression have increased dramatically during the past half century in the United States despite—or perhaps partly because of—an armamentarium of new medications (10). Epilepsy is a chronic disorder with acute symptoms, falling between these two poles. Complementary and alternative medicine may have its greatest benefits by helping patients improve their lifestyle and reduce their stress, thereby promoting physical and mental health, which could reduce seizures and improve quality of life. These are all enormous potential benefits for people with epilepsy.

Complementary and alternative medicine and MM must define the benefits and risks of their therapies. Neither has done a good job here. In epilepsy care, quantifying outcome is difficult because epilepsy is so much more than seizures. It is how seizures and their aftermath impact a person, how the diagnosis and stigma affect a person's life, and how medications affect the individual's mind and body. Even seizures are not so easy to quantify since they often occur randomly and with variable frequency. Seizure occurrence is influenced by lifestyle factors such as sleep deprivation, stress, alcohol use, hormones, and medical illness. Humans are terrible at seeing things as random. Our minds are wired to find patterns by linking temporal associations with cause and effect (11). The person who links the eating of mushrooms with vomiting an hour later will survive and pass along those genes. Those genes also curse humans with false patterns. Once we identify a pattern, our confirmation bias finds supportive evidence and ignores or rationalizes refuting evidence. Our desire for answers far exceeds our ability for humility. People want to know *why*. Why do I have epilepsy? What caused my seizure on this day? We often cannot answer these questions. False answers are worse than admitting ignorance since false answers stop people from looking.

There are biases in MM and CAM. Job security, financial rewards, and ego can influence health care workers, hospitals, companies, health care administrators, and basic scientists, as well as CAM therapists. There is tremendous pressure to maintain a dysfunctional status quo when the status quo supports you. As Upton Sinclair (12) said so eloquently, "It is difficult to get a man to understand something when his job depends on not understanding it" (p. 109). Health care—MM and CAM—employs a lot of people.

Many in MM see their discipline as the product of science, while CAM rests on biased anecdotes and observations. However, doctors often exaggerate the quality of the evidence and confuse belief for data. Even the DB-PC-RT, the pinnacle of evidence, can easily be misinterpreted, falsely extrapolated, and abused. Large DB-PC-RTs can yield statistically significant results of uncertain clinical import. Consider a man taking 400 mg per day of lamotrigine and experiencing 4 complex partial seizures per month. His neurologist adds 3,600 mg of gabapentin, and his seizure frequency declines to 3 per month, a 25% reduction. The same effect in 30 patients yields statistical significance. However, has the additional medication done more harm than benefit? It did not change driving status. The man traded 1.5 minutes of seizure freedom for 43,000 minutes per month of increased tiredness and dizziness and an 8-pound weight gain. Statistics say this extra medicine is helpful, but common sense says it hurts.

Numbers are not always what they appear to be. Patient reports are often unreliable, as absence, complex partial, and tonic-clonic seizures impair consciousness, and many patients and witnesses are unaware they occurred. In an epilepsy monitoring unit, only 63% of patients recalled having had a seizure. One of our patients activated her vagus nerve stimulator with a magnet during her aura. She proceeded to have a complex partial seizure but was convinced the magnet stopped the seizure because the last thing she recalled was using the magnet. Does the magnet abort seizures in some people with epilepsy? Almost 15 years after approval by the Food and Drug Administration (FDA), the answer is that we do not know. How does one distinguish the role of the intervention from the natural time course of the seizure? It can be done, but it is a challenging study.

How reproducible are DB-PC-RTs? Jonah Lehrer (14) highlights multiple examples where these studies, which led to FDA approval for medications, somehow faded with time and repetition. For example, the efficacy of the second-generation antipsychotic drugs (e.g., aripiprazole, quetiapine, and olanzapine) appeared much greater than the first-generation antipsychotic drugs during initial DB-PC-RT, but in subsequent studies, their efficacy declined. The declines were over 50% in some studies. Similarly, one study of antidepressants found a greater than 50% decline in efficacy over time. The effect is not limited to psychiatric medications but also includes the benefits of vitamins and cardiac stents. The bias of journals to publish selectively positive findings likely accounts for some of this, but another factor may be our ability to unconsciously or consciously bias results, even when we are supposed to be blinded. For example, studies of acupuncture in Asian countries are much more likely to find positive results than studies of acupuncture in Western countries. A telling example was a review of 49 highly cited original studies published in 3 major clinical journals in which an intervention was effective (15). Of these, 16% were contradicted by subsequent studies, 16% found effects that were stronger than those of subsequent studies, 44% were replicated, and 24% remained largely unchallenged. Thus, of those in which replication was done, 41% were either contradicted or found a significantly smaller effect than originally reported. None showed a significantly larger effect. Why? Is there something deeply flawed in the scientific method, or is it just the people who use this method?

Epilepsy is a chronic disorder, but DB-PC-RT studies on medications for FDA approval typically occur in 6 months or less. Common side effects such as fatigue, stomach discomfort, and dizziness allegedly improve with time—or is it that people just get used to feeling badly? As the doctor gradually increases the dose, problems recur but later resolve. Patients on the same drug for years often deny any side effects, but when their medication is stopped, they note an incredible improvement in energy, mental clarity, and mood. Doctors reassure patients that there are "no long-term side effects," without rigorous scientific data. Even worse, doctors may extrapolate from short-term DB-PC-RT studies to assure patients about long-term safety.

Approval by the FDA can open Pandora's box. Consider antiepileptic drug (AED) use in psychiatry. Gabapentin was approved to treat partial epilepsy. The indication was later extended to include some pain disorders but never any psychiatric disorders. Studies funded by the drug company supported its use in bipolar disorder. Among 29 studies on gabapentin for bipolar disorder, 4 were randomized trials, and 2 were crossover trials; most were uncontrolled. These 29 trials were cited more than 1,000 times in 429 medical articles (16). Well-controlled studies found that gabapentin is not effective for bipolar disorder (17–18). Gabapentin is widely prescribed for bipolar, anxiety, depression, and other psychiatric disorders. In 2004, Warner-Lambert paid $430 million in fines to settle criminal and civil charges for improperly promoting off-label use of the drug. Gabapentin is the tip of the AED-use-in-psychiatry iceberg, as many other AEDs are used without scientific data and sometimes cause behavioral side effects.

The controversy surrounding generic drugs provides valuable lessons. Brand-name drugs are expensive, and insurance companies, hospitals, and patients without health insurance want less expensive, generic drugs. Where do the doctors stand? Scientifically, we lack adequate data to decide. For a person with well-controlled epilepsy who often drives, a single seizure can be deadly. Generic drugs must have a confidence interval for bioequivalence, but this allows for greater differences in blood levels (19). Simulating pairs of generic AED combinations, the total drug exposures differed by more than 15% for 17% of pairs, and peak concentrations varied by more than 15% in 39% of pairs. The AEDs with low bioavailability and solubility (e.g., oxcarbazepine) have the greatest variance in bioequivalence (20). Data suggest that the change from brand to generic medication may not be benign (21). Yet understanding cause and effect is complex. If the change from brand-name to generic AEDs is associated with increased seizures or side effects, does that prove that the generic drug is responsible? No. Another rarely considered explanation is that brand-name drugs enjoy a greater placebo effect. In a study of placebo pain medications, patients reported experiencing much greater pain relief when they were told the "drug" cost $2.50 per pill than when it cost $0.10 per pill (22). The connection of expectation and outcome is a weapon and curse. An effective drug can be rendered ineffective if it is delivered with the expectation of failure, and a placebo can be dramatically effective when offered with the promise of great success.

In health care, two powerful, invisible, widespread, and dangerous biases are the desire to help and the need to be helped. Patients seek care to hear answers and receive therapies. They do not want to hear "the cause is unknown" and "an effective therapy does not exist." Practitioners are trained to give answers and prescribe therapies. It is much easier to treat than to explain that there is no treatment.

Most practitioners are unable to question the evidence for what they do. Confirmation bias surrounds us. Despite its limitations, the scientific method remains our best tool to gather objective information and translate that data into better health care outcomes. The Appendix (Levels of Evidence in Medical Science) summarizes the different types of data used to support a test or therapy. Richard Feynman (1) raised the following strange paradox: in our scientific age, we have difficulty understanding how witch doctors ever existed and how healers in the Middle Ages used rhinoceros horn powder to increase potency, yet we are surrounded by the same phenomenon cloaked in different garments. For Feynman, reflexology's location of a pituitary spot at the center of the big-toe print whorl rests on no greater evidence than witchcraft.

What is the quality of the data to support CAM in epilepsy? It is limited. We lack data to establish the efficacy of most CAM in epilepsy. No well-controlled, adequately powered study has assessed chiropractic, craniosacral, acupuncture, massage, meditation, or any other CAM therapies for epilepsy. Lack of good data leaves the door open but should not support any therapy. The Cochrane Central Library of Controlled Trials performed meta-analyses of acupuncture and yoga in epilepsy and concluded that there are insufficient data to show any benefits (23–24). However, the study was unable to find data to disprove the benefits of acupuncture and yoga. One could also hypothesize that vitamin C or magnetic necklaces can reduce seizure activity, but without data, it is impossible to endorse either therapy. Furthermore, "natural" does not always mean safe. Many vitamin supplements were considered "risk free," but studies have found that natural supplements of antioxidants may actually increase the risk of some cancers (25).

Many patients and families face the challenge of ongoing seizures or side effects with MM. Complementary and alternative medicine offers natural approaches that appear safe and are supported by their patients and practitioners. What to do? As with MM, we remain humble about what we know and what we do not know. We should be skeptical of therapies that lack any theoretical basis. We should be more skeptical of those who profess certainty but lack data. Those who "know" that their MM or CAM therapy works but lack DB-PC-RT data are fooling themselves at best and fooling you at worst. The more practitioners "believe," the more bias infects their minds. Our goal is to apply the skepticism of science to explore the range of CAM reported to be helpful in treating epilepsy.

SOME CAM DISCIPLINES WITH LITTLE OR NO COVERAGE

Our choice of topics reflects both the theoretical nature as well as the supportive data. For some CAM therapies, neither the theoretical basis nor the published studies provide sufficient support to include in this volume. This does not mean that they or other CAM therapies not discussed here are ineffective. Rather, we are unable to identify potential mechanisms or supportive evidence for these therapies. Examples include chiropractic and osteopathic therapies which receive brief coverage as well as oxygen therapies which are not covered beyond this section.

Chiropractic therapy is a well-established discipline used extensively to treat neck and back pain. The scientific literature strongly supports the effectiveness of chiropractic therapy to treat these disorders affecting muscles, ligaments, nerves, and bones. Chiropractic therapy is also used to treat headache and fibromyalgia, although the evidence to support its effectiveness is less than for neck and back pain. Since headache can result from muscle tension or from cervical spine pain radiation, improvement in headache after chiropractic therapy has a clear theoretical basis. There are no controlled medical studies supporting chiropractic therapy for epilepsy care. Case reports and small series report patients in whom chiropractic therapy was associated with improved seizure control. In one case, chiropractic manipulation was applied during a seizure, and the seizure abated. Although these cases are suggestive, none are based on either randomized or placebo-controlled trials. Most seizures last less than 2 minutes, so any therapy or observation during a seizure is likely to be associated with seizure cessation. The theoretical basis for improved seizure control by chiropractic therapy is increased blood flow to the brain. The vertebral arteries that supply the lower brain pass through the transverse foramina of multiple cervical vertebrae. Thus, if there was a problem with blood flow in the vertebral arteries caused, for example, by narrowing of these foramina, a widening of these passages could improve blood flow to the brain. The problem is that there is no evidence that chiropractic therapy can improve blood flow in the vertebral arteries. Further, there is no evidence that improving blood flow in a vertebral artery (e.g., with anticoagulants or other agents) can improve seizure control.

Osteopathic therapy has a rich history dating back to 1884, with an initial focus on bones. The current discipline extends to structural integrity of all body regions, including the brain. Osteopathic medicine closely examines the ways in which abnormalities in the body's function or structure cause pain and disorders. Osteopathic doctors (DOs) receive education and training that parallels that of medical doctors. Osteopathic doctors care for patients in private practices and academic medical centers alongside medical doctors with equal expertise and similar diagnostic and therapeutic approaches. However, there is another group of DOs who primarily assess the inherent primary respiratory mechanism and the inherent brain rhythm to identify abnormalities that may cause epilepsy. Gentle palpitation is used to diagnose these abnormalities, and "appropriate techniques" are used to correct the problem (26). There is no evidence of an inherent brain rhythm that can be identified by palpating the head. There is no evidence that one can modify this mysterious rhythm by appropriate techniques. Some of these CAM DOs believe that birth trauma, minor head injuries, and immunizations commonly cause epilepsy (26). There is extensive evidence that these factors are not common causes of epilepsy. Thus, the mainstream DOs provide care to people with epilepsy based on medical science, while the CAM group of DOs provide diagnoses and treatments whose basis remains undefined (at least to us) and which we can identify no objective data to support. We will not discuss them further.

Enhancing the delivery of oxygen to the brain also forms the theoretical basis for other CAM epilepsy therapies: rebreathing and hyperbaric oxygen. The rebreathing technique forms the core therapy used by the Institutes for the Achievement of Human Potential. Having patients intermittently rebreath their exhaled carbon dioxide raises blood and brain carbon dioxide levels to dilate cerebral blood vessels, stimulate respiratory drive, and acidify the blood. Overall, this facilitates release of oxygen from hemoglobin. Together, these factors are considered to increase the delivery of oxygen to the brain and thereby help to control seizures (27–29). However, increasing carbon dioxide concentrations shifts the oxygen-hemoglobin dissociation curve to the right and lowers the oxygen saturation of hemoglobin. There are no data that people with epilepsy experience impaired delivery of oxygen to their brain or that increasing blood oxygen levels to above normal improves seizure control. If oxygen therapy benefits people with epilepsy, oxygen via nasal prongs can be more easily administered with much less effort. Thus, we are left with a therapy that has no solid theoretical foundation and no objective evidence of efficacy. Hyperbaric oxygen is a standard medical therapy for decompression sickness (the "bends," which can affect scuba divers who ascend too rapidly), diabetic wound healing, and some other disorders. Its use for various neurologic disorders such as multiple sclerosis, cerebral palsy, and epilepsy is not supported by scientific data. Indeed, one double-blind trial of hyperbaric oxygen therapy for cerebral palsy found a greater benefit from placebo than active therapy (30). This highlights the power of placebos (both treatment groups benefited). Without the placebo arm, one would falsely conclude that the treatment led to the improvement.

COMPLEMENTARY AND ALTERNATIVE MEDICINE: COMING OF AGE

Some CAM is effective and is now part of MM. Examples include the ketogenic and modified Atkins diet. Some areas are supported by independent studies, but DB-PC-RTs are lacking. These include the following: (a) behavioral techniques (e.g., Andrews/Reiter program, discussed in Chapter 6) that seek to identify provocative factors or settings that make seizures more likely and teach patients to minimize or avoid these; and (b) various methods of stress reduction (e.g., exercise, yoga, elimination of stressful lifestyle issues). Other types of CAM are supported by animal studies and/or limited human data (e.g., some herbal treatments and neuroelectroencephalographic feedback, discussed in Chapter 6).

The expansion of CAM is visible in governmental policies, medical literature, and patient use. The incorporation of CAM into health care varies tremendously in Western societies. In Germany, the use of medicinal herbs is regulated by legislation and covered by health insurers. Data on CAM are greatly expanding. Between 2001 and 2011, entries about "alternative medicine" on PubMed, a U.S. National Library of Medicine online listing of articles in selected medical journals, increased from 46,800 to 195,700. In 1997, more than one third of the U.S. population used a CAM therapy, and 67.6% used at least one CAM therapy in their life. Lifetime use steadily increased with age (31).

This book is intended to provide an overview of CAM for epilepsy. We remain open to the possibility that significant advancements can be achieved in reducing seizures and medication side effects as well as in improvement of quality of life through CAM. This is our attempt to better understand the range of the CAM therapies, to explain what those therapies involve, and to assess the evidence for their safety and efficacy. We hope to leverage some of the skepticism of science with the holistic, preventive, and positivistic views of CAM. Health care is a partnership of patient and practitioner, of prevention and therapy, and of MM and CAM. No one approach, therapy, or model will work for all people or illnesses. We must accept our ignorance, acknowledge the complexity of biologic systems, focus sharply on our bias, and embrace new approaches that are shown to be safe and effective.

REFERENCES

1. Feynman RP. *Surely You're Joking, Mr. Feynman!: Adventures of a Curious Character.* New York, NY: W.W. Norton & Company; 1997.
2. *Living With Epilepsy: Report of a Roper Poll of Patients on Quality of Life.* New York, NY: Roper Organization, Inc., 1992.
3. Devinsky O, Penry JK. Quality of life in epilepsy: the clinician's perspective. *Epilepsia.* 1993;34(S4):S4–S7.
4. Begley CE, Famulari M, Annegers JF, et al. The cost of epilepsy in the United States: an estimate from population-based clinical and survey data. *Epilepsia.* 2000;41(3):342–51.
5. Sieveking EH. *Epilepsy and Epileptic Seizures.* London: Churchill Livingstone; 1858.
6. Kim C, Kwok YS. Navajo use of native healers. *Arch Intern Med.* 1998;158:2245–2249.
7. Coulehan JL. Navaho Indian medicine: implications for healing. *J Fam Pract.* 1980;10:55–61.
8. Gladwell M. *Blink: The Power of Thinking Without Thinking.* New York, NY: Little, Brown and Company; 2005.
9. Servan-Schreiber D. *Anticancer: A New Way of Life.* New York, NY: Viking Adult; 2009.
10. Whitaker R. *Anatomy of an Epidemic: Magic Bullets, Psychiatric Drugs, and the Astonishing Rise of Mental Illness in America.* New York, NY: Crown; 2010.
11. Mlodinow L. *The Drunkard's Walk: How Randomness Rules Our Lives.* New York, NY: Vintage Books; 2008.

12. Sinclair U. *I, Candidate for Governor: And How I Got Licked.* Los Angeles, CA: University of California Press; 1994.
13. Dubois JM, Boylan LS, Shiyko M, et al. Seizure prediction and recall. *Epilepsy Behav.* 2010;18(1-2):106–109.
14. Lehrer J. The truth wears off: is there something wrong with the scientific method? http://www.newyorker.com/reporting/2010/12/13/101213fa_fact_lehrer?currentPage=all. Accessed October 23, 2011.
15. Ioannidis JP. Contradicted and initially stronger effects in highly cited clinical research. *JAMA.* 2005;294:218–228.
16. Yan J. Drug-marketing excesses fund medication-education campaign. *Psychiatr News.* 2009;44(12):7.
17. Vieta E, Manuel Goikolea J, Martínez-Arán A, et al. A double-blind, randomized, placebo-controlled, prophylaxis study of adjunctive gabapentin for bipolar disorder. *J Clin Psychiatry.* 2006;67:473–477.
18. Pande AC, Crockatt JG, Janney CA, et al. Gabapentin in bipolar disorder: a placebo-controlled trial of adjunctive therapy. Gabapentin Bipolar Disorder Study Group. *Bipolar Disord.* 2000;2:249–255.
19. Heaney DC, Sander JW. Antiepileptic drugs: generic versus branded treatments. *Lancet Neurol.* 2007;6:465–468.
20. Krauss GL, Caffo B, Chang YT, et al. Assessing bioequivalence of generic antiepilepsy drugs. *Ann Neurol.* 2011;70:221–228.
21. Labiner DM, Paradis PE, Manjunath R, et al. Generic antiepileptic drugs and associated medical resource utilization in the United States. *Neurology.* 2010;74(20):1566–1574.
22. Ariely D. *Predictably Irrational: The Hidden Forces That Shape our Decisions.* New York, NY: HarperCollins; 2008.
23. Cheuk DK, Wong V. Acupuncture for epilepsy. *Cochrane Database of Systematic Reviews* 2008, Issue 4. Art. No.: CD005062.
24. Ramaratnam S, Sridharan K. Yoga for epilepsy. *Cochrane Database of Systematic Reviews* 2000, Issue 2. Art. No.: CD001524.
25. Greenlee H, Kwan ML, Kushi LH, et al. Antioxidant supplement use after breast cancer diagnosis and mortality in the Life After Cancer Epidemiology (LACE) corhort. *Cancer.* 2012:118:2048–58.
26. Fryman, VM. The osteopathic approach to children with seizure disorders. In: Devinsky O, Schachter S, Pacia S, eds. *Complementary and Alternative Therapies for Epilepsy.* New York, NY: Demos Medical Publishing; 2005:273–84.
27. Schmidt CF. The influence of cerebral blood flow in respiration. I. The respiratory responses to change in cerebral blood flow. II. The gaseous metabolism of the brain. III. The interplay of factors concerned in the relation of respiration. *Am J Physiol.* 1928;84:202,223,242.
28. Lennox WG, Cobb S. Relation of certain physio-chemical processes to epileptiform seizures. *Am J Psychiatry.* 1929;8:837–847.
29. Fay T. The therapeutic effect of dehydration on epileptic patients. *Arch Neurol Psychiatry.* 1930; 23: 920–945.
30. Hardy P, Collet JP, Goldberg J, et al. Neuropsychological effects of hyperbaric oxygen therapy in cerebral palsy. *Dev Med Child Neurol.* 2002;44:436–446.
31. Kessler RC, Davis RB, Foster DF, et al. Long-term trends in the use of complementary and alternative medical therapies in the United States. *Ann Intern Med.* 2001;135:262–268.

2

Herbal Remedies

Nearly 1 in 3 people with epilepsy (PWE) continues to have seizures despite taking prescription seizure medications (AEDs) (1–2). Many PWE experience troubling side effects from AEDs. Still, others suffer from epilepsy-related conditions such as depression, anxiety, sleep disorders, or migraine headaches, which are examples of the comorbidities of epilepsy. It is therefore not surprising that PWEs often look for other solutions to control seizures and ways to reduce AED-related side effects or the symptoms of comorbidities, as discussed throughout this book.

Herbal remedies originate from plants and are often called "botanicals." They are among the most commonly tried forms of complementary and alternative therapies used by PWE (see Figure 2.1 for categories of such therapies) (3). They are classified by the National Center for Complementary and Alternative Medicine (NCCAM) as belonging to the domain of biologically based practices, which generally includes substances found in nature, such as herbs, foods, vitamins, and animal compounds. Herbal remedies are often an integral part of medical systems recognized by the National Center for Complementary and Alternative Medicine, such as homeopathy, naturopathy, Ayurveda, and traditional Chinese medicine (TCM), each of which encompasses a comprehensive system of diagnostics and therapeutics that include herbal remedies. Biologically based CAM treatments can also be obtained by U.S. consumers in the form of dietary supplements (as defined in Figure 2.2), without any associated diagnostic or treatment plan as directed by a practitioner (4).

At present, there are no published clinical trials on herbal remedies for the treatment of epilepsy that definitively demonstrate safety, tolerability, or effectiveness, including herbs used in TCM (5). However, approaches for overcoming the methodological shortcomings of past herbal studies are emerging, as are new findings from scientific laboratories on the actions of herbal remedies on brain cells and experimentally induced seizures. These developments are likely to spur on additional research and enhance the quality and outcomes of clinical trials in the future.

Figure 2.1   Categories of complementary and alternative health practices recognized by the National Center for Complementary and Alternative Medicine.

Categories	Examples
Natural products	Herbal medicines (botanicals), vitamins, minerals
Mind & body medicine	Meditation, yoga, acupuncture, deep-breathing exercises, guided imagery, hypnotherapy, progressive relaxation, qigong, tai chi
Manipulative & body-based practices	Spinal manipulation, massage
Other	Movement therapies, traditional healers, energy therapies, whole medical systems (Ayurvedic medicine, traditional Chinese medicine, homeopathy, naturopathy)

Adapted from The National Center for Complementary and Alternative Medicine (3).

This chapter discusses the frequency of use of herbal remedies by PWE as well as potential benefits and problems associated with their use. Several traditional medical systems that use herbal remedies are described, and the regulation of herbal remedies in the United States and safety issues are highlighted.

SCOPE OF USE OF HERBAL REMEDIES

General population

Herbal remedies and other nature-based therapies were the primary form of treatment for patients around the world for centuries. Over the past century, the use of herbal remedies by doctors in the developed world (who practice what is generally called "Western medicine") has gradually, and nearly completely, been

Figure 2.2   Definition of a dietary supplement from the U.S. Food and Drug Administration.

A dietary supplement is a product taken by mouth that contains a dietary ingredient intended to supplement the diet.
The dietary ingredients in these products may include vitamins, minerals, herbs, or other botanicals; amino acids; & substances such as enzymes, organ tissues, glandulars, & metabolites.
Dietary supplements can also be extracts or concentrates & may be found in many forms, such as tablets, capsules, softgels, gelcaps, liquids, or powders.
Dietary supplements can also take other forms, such as a bar. If they do, information on their label must not represent the product as a conventional food or a sole item of a meal or diet.

Adapted from the U.S. Food and Drug Administration (4).

replaced by single-compound pharmaceutical drugs, such as AEDs. This trend has occurred at the same time that government regulatory agencies, such as the U.S. Food and Drug Administration (FDA), have established increasingly strict standards for manufacturing and conducting laboratory and clinical tests on pharmaceuticals, thereby enhancing the confidence that patients and their physicians have in the quality, safety, and effectiveness of prescription drugs. By contrast, as will be further discussed, the regulation of herbal remedies, even in developed countries like the United States, does not ensure the safety and quality of these products in the marketplace.

Healthy persons as well as patients with chronic neurologic illnesses that respond poorly or incompletely to conventional treatments (e.g., epilepsy, back pain, anxiety, depression, headaches, and fibromyalgia) may use herbal remedies for a variety of reasons (6). Some people prefer natural treatments to "artificial" or "synthetic" drugs, assuming that natural treatments are better and safer. Others may believe that alternative health care providers give them more control over their health care decisions. A U.S. survey in 2007 of over 23,000 adults and 9,000 children selected from the general population found that nearly 1 in 3 adults and 1 in 8 children reported using CAM therapies (7). Among these, natural products, such as herbal remedies, were used by nearly half the adults who acknowledged using CAM therapies. The most frequently tried herbal remedies were echinacea, flaxseed, and ginseng. The costs to U.S. consumers for natural products in 2007 were estimated to be $14.8 billion, about one third the amount spent by consumers on prescription drugs (8).

People with epilepsy

A number of studies have shown that adult and pediatric PWE often use CAM therapies (see Table 2.1) (9). According to these studies, up to 1 in 2 adults and 1 in 3 children with epilepsy have tried one or more CAM therapies. However, less than half do so in order to control seizures; the most often-cited reason is general health maintenance.

A number of these studies identified specific natural products taken by PWE. Ekstein and Schachter (9) analyzed these findings and found that the 3 most frequently taken products overall were ginseng (reported by 17%), *Ginkgo biloba* (16%), and St. John's wort (13%). These findings suggest that some PWE may take these products to reduce symptoms of epilepsy-related comorbidities because these particular herbal remedies are often taken for symptoms of anxiety, depression, and memory deficits, respectively, which commonly occur in PWE (10). Therefore, the herbal remedies taken by PWE may be clues to possible side effects from AEDs or symptoms of possible comorbidities.

The herbal remedies documented in these studies varied. For example, one survey of PWE found that ginseng, St. John's wort, melatonin, *Ginkgo biloba*, garlic, and black cohosh were the most frequently taken herbal medicines and dietary supplements, whereas another found that garlic, *Ginkgo biloba*, soy, melatonin, and kava were most often taken (11–12).

Table 2.1 Publications Reporting on Use of Complementary and Alternative Medicine in Countries With a Western-Style Medical System

Studied Population	% Using CAM	Associations	Doctor's Knowledge	Most Used CAM (in Descending Order, Where Known)	Reason for Use	Outcome Measures	Most Used Nonvitamin, Nonmineral Natural Products (in Descending Order, Where Known)
465 adults with epilepsy from 9 regions in the United States	31%, within previous year	Associated with high-school education or less; no influence of age, sex, seizure type	33%	Ginkgo biloba, vitamins (55%), relaxation (45%), ginseng, St. John's wort	13% epilepsy (relaxation, vitamins, herbals, homeopathy); 28% general health/cold prevention; 11% mood difficulties; 5% cognition; 4% fatigue	NA	Ginkgo biloba (81% of users, 63% used it for cognition); ginseng (44% of users); St. John's wort (used by 7% of patients, 53% for mood & 24% for fatigue)
92 adults with epilepsy in Ohio (United States)	24%	No significant association with education level, sex, ethnicity, age	31%	Massage (50%), herbs/supplements (41%), music therapy, meditation, art therapy, aromatherapy, acupuncture	2% epilepsy (massage, acupuncture & meditation); pain; muscle tension; stress; low energy; cold; depression	NA	4 ginseng, 3 St. John's wort, 3 melatonin, 3 Ginkgo biloba, 1 garlic, 1 black cohosh
198 children with active epilepsy in Norway	11.6%	Additional neurologic deficits	NA	Homeopathy	NA	NA	NA

115 children with epilepsy in Israel (compared with children with ADHD & control)	32%	In general: higher education, prior use for current use; for epilepsy & ADHD: longer disease duration, less satisfaction with conventional therapy	NA	Dietary interventions most and also homeopathy, biofeedback, acupuncture, Reike, reflexology, Shiatsu, chiropractic (in all groups)	NA	NA	NA
425 adults with epilepsy in Arizona (United States)	44% for epilepsy, 42% for other conditions	No association with education level	93% would tell	Prayer, stress management, botanicals, chiropractic (specifically for epilepsy)	44% epilepsy; 42% other conditions	Stress management, yoga, and botanicals subjectively most beneficial; 43% using botanicals for epilepsy had increased seizure frequency; 3 had major side effects (intracranial hemorrhage with ephedra)	General/epilepsy use: 76/13 garlic, 157/12 ginkgo, 64/10 soy, 40/11 melatonin, 22/10 kava, 159/8 ginseng, 147/9 St. John's wort, 89/9 echinacea, 68/3 cranberry, 40/5 goldenseal, 24/7 grape seed, 21/4 black cohosh, 33/4 valerian, 14/3 saw palmetto, 7/7 evening primrose, 12/2 licorice, 7/4 hops, 3/2 black haw

(continued)

Table 2.1 Publications Reporting on Use of Complementary and Alternative Medicine in Countries With a Western-Style Medical System (*continued*)

Studied Population	% Using CAM	Associations	Doctor's Knowledge	Most Used CAM (in Descending Order, Where Known)	Reason for Use	Outcome Measures	Most Used Nonvitamin, Nonmineral Natural Products (in Descending Order, Where Known)
187 adults with epilepsy in San Francisco area (United States)	56%	No association with seizure frequency or with having adverse events from AED	68%	Vitamin or mineral supplements	3% epilepsy or AED adverse events; general health; supplementing diet; physician's recommendation	NA (19% used products with CYP450 activity and 14% used potentially epileptogenic agents)	Garlic, echinacea, St. John's wort, ephedra, ginseng, ginkgo, evening primrose
350 children with epilepsy neurologic conditions (60% had epilepsy) in Pennsylvania (United States)	28% of children with epilepsy (37% of all conditions)	Diagnosed for less than 1 year	69%	NA	NA	87% overall felt CAM was effective and similar to conventional therapy; 40% knew possible side effects	NA

Sample	Prevalence	Association	Percentage	CAM types	Use for epilepsy	Outcome	Specific herbs
377 adults with epilepsy in Manchester, United Kingdom	34.6%	Higher education	37%	NA	11.1% epilepsy	No significant effect on seizure frequency; CAM was cheap	NA
228 adults with epilepsy in midwest United States	39%	No association with education level	49%	Prayer/spirituality, megavitamins, chiropractic, stress management	57 (25%) epilepsy: 33 prayer/spirituality; 14 megavitamins; 11 chiropractic; 11 stress management	Subjective benefit of 74% of 57; only few side effects	10 cranberry, 8 black cohosh, 7 echinacea, 6 melatonin, 4 garlic, 4 grape seed, 4 soy, 4 St. John's wort, 4 valerian, 3 evening primrose, 2 *Ginkgo biloba*, 2 ginseng, 1 black haw
671 adults with neurologic conditions in Ireland (189 with epilepsy)	47.6% of people with epilepsy (63.3% of all conditions)	NA	25% for all conditions	Massage, acupuncture, vitamins, reflexology, yoga, evening primrose/starflower oil, chiropractic, homeopathy (for all conditions)	NA	Most had subjective benefit; annual cost was 1170.32 euro	97 evening primrose/starflower oil, 24 marijuana, 16 St. John's wort, 16 *Ginkgo biloba*, Udo's Oil, fish oil, black cohosh, echinacea, bone meal, coenzyme Q10

(continued)

Table 2.1 Publications Reporting on Use of Complementary and Alternative Medicine in Countries With a Western-Style Medical System (*continued*)

Studied Population	% Using CAM	Associations	Doctor's Knowledge	Most Used CAM (in Descending Order, Where Known)	Reason for Use	Outcome Measures	Most Used Nonvitamin, Nonmineral Natural Products (in Descending Order, Where Known)
187 adults with epilepsy at UCSF medical center (United States)	56% (current use)	Partial epilepsy and race (white); no association with sex, age, level of education, income, duration of epilepsy, or seizure frequency	71%	Multivitamins and minerals, folic acid, ginseng, *Ginkgo biloba*, glucosamine and chondroitin, St. John's wort, black cohosh, echinacea, evening primrose, ephedra, caffeine, melatonin, milk thistle, omega-3, kava, skullcap, valerian, grapefruit juice, glutamine, clover/nettles, parsley leaf, DHEA, coenzyme Q10, ginger, fish oil, garlic, grape seed, L-lysine	6 epilepsy (kava, skullcap, valerian, folic acid, vitamin B_6, vitamin E, multivitamins, minerals); 35 general health; 13 physician's recommendation; 13 improve bone density; 10 increase energy; 10 boost immune system; 7 improve memory	9 patients reported adverse events that they attributed to these products; none reported aggravation of seizures; 88% of patients spent less than $50 a month, & only 5% spent more than $100	4 ginseng, 4 *Ginkgo biloba*, 4 glucosamine and chondroitin, 3 St. John's wort, 2 black cohosh, 2 echinacea, 2 evening primrose, 2 ephedra, 2 caffeine, 2 melatonin, 2 milk thistle, 2 omega-3, 1 kava, 1 skullcap, 1 valerian, 1 grapefruit juice, 1 glutamine, 1 clover/nettles, 1 parsley leaf, 1 DHEA, 1 coenzyme Q10, 1 ginger, 1 fish oil, 1 garlic, 1 grape seed, 1 L-lysine

Abbreviations: ADHD, attention-deficit hyperactivity disorder; AED, antiepileptic drug; CAM, complementary and alternative medicine; DHEA, dehydroepiandrosterone; NA, not applicable; UCSF, University of California–San Francisco. Reprinted with permission from Ekstein and Schachter (9).

A Medline search on the 35 products found in the surveys cited in Table 2.1 was conducted to evaluate their main uses, adverse events, potential for drug interactions, and known or presumed effects on seizures and on AEDs (see Table 2.2) (9). For example, ginseng, *Ginkgo biloba*, and St. John's wort have been anecdotally reported to improve *as well as to worsen* seizures, depending on the part of the plant that is ingested or the extraction method. Also, the authors cautioned that *Ginkgo biloba* and St. John's wort might interact with AEDs that are metabolized by the liver, which may cause potentially unsafe fluctuations in AED serum concentrations.

HERBAL REMEDIES AND TRADITIONAL MEDICAL SYSTEMS

Herbal remedies have been used to treat seizures for centuries and, consequently, have been a major part of traditional medical systems, some of which still exist today. For example, the use of herbal remedies for seizures dates back to 6000 BC in India and to 3000 BC in China. Indeed, the 2 oldest documented medical systems are from China (TCM) and India (Ayurveda). Each of these systems has theories about the diagnosis and treatment of epilepsy that guide the selection of herbal remedies and other treatments. However, these theories are not understandable in the context of the biomedical framework taught to U.S. medical students. Epilepsy specialists at U.S. medical centers may therefore find the seizure classification system used in these traditional systems, along with the rationale for choosing treatments, to be confusing. Other systems that use herbal remedies, such as homeopathy (addressed later in this chapter) and naturopathy, have been elaborated on more recently but still may not be congruent with the theories of medicine taught in U.S. medical schools (13).

Traditional Chinese medicine

The role of herbal remedies in TCM is well described and documented (14). The use of such products in China for epilepsy was first documented in a book called *The Yellow Emperor's Classic of Internal Medicine (Huang Di Nei Ching)*, which was written more than 2,200 years ago (15). Today, forms of TCM are practiced widely within and outside of China and are sometimes financially supported by government health authorities. In Japan, for example, herbal remedies—called Kampo medicines—are reimbursed by the "National Health system."

Herbal remedies traditionally used to treat convulsions in Asia include Chai-Hu-Long-Ku-Mu-Li-Tan, a mixture of extracts from 13 herbal medicines; *Gastrodia elata*; *Uncaria rhynchophylla*; *Menispermum dauricum*; Shitei-To, a mixture of extracts from 3 medicinal herbs (*Shitei* [kaki calyx, calyx of *Diospyros kaki* L.f.], *Shokyo* [zingiberis rhizoma, rhizome of *Zingiber officinale* Roscoe], and *Choji* [caryophylli flos, flower bud of *Syzygium aromaticum* L.]); *Qingyangshen*, a mixture of radish and pepper (which contains the alkaloid piperine); Kanbaku-taiso-to, a mixture of 3 herbal drugs (Glycyrrhizae Radix, Tritici Semen and

Table 2.2 Characteristics of Natural Products Used by People With Epilepsy in Countries With a Western-Based Type of Medical System[a]

Product	Main Current Medical Uses	Main Adverse Events & Interactions	Overall Estimated Extent of Use in PWEs[b]	Possible Effects in Epilepsy	Potential Risks for PWEs
Black cohosh (*Cimicifuga racemosa*)	Ameliorates menopausal symptoms	Possible hepatotoxicity	4%	NR	NR
Black haw (*Viburnum prunifolium*)	Spasmolytic; sedative; antiasthmatic	NR	<1%	NR	NR
Bone meal	Calcium supplementation (not used recently)	Possible prion infection		NR	NR Seizures secondary to lead poisoning
Caffeine	Stimulant; antinociceptive	Sympathomimetic & GI symptoms	<1%	NR	Associated with seizures; may interact with CBZ
Chondroitin	Antiarthritis; antiarthralgia	GI symptoms, hypersensitivity, possible anticoagulation (increased INR with warfarin)	<1%	NR	NR
(Red) clover (*Trifolium pretense*)	Ameliorates menopausal symptoms	Possibly inhibits aromatase & extrahepatic CYP1A1, 1B1; may increase INR when taken with warfarin	<1%	NR	NR

Coenzyme Q10	Antioxidant; ameliorates CHF & neurodegenerative disorders	May increase risk of bleeding in warfarin users	<1%	May improve seizures in neurologic mitochondrial diseases	NR
Cranberry	Prevents UTI; cardioprotector; anticancer; antioxidant	GI intolerance, weight gain, possibly thrombocytopenia & increase in INR in combination with warfarin	9%	NR	NR Inhibited P450 system in vitro but not in vivo
DHEA	Hormonal replacement therapy in elderly women & men	No adverse events; induces CYP2B6	<1%	NR No effect in animals	Possibly associated with seizures
Echinacea	Enhances immune system functions	Hypersensitivity, GI disturbance, hepatotoxicity with prolonged use; mild effect on CYP3A4 & CYP1A2	11%	NR	NR
Ephedra	Induces weight loss; stimulant	HTN, tachycardia, stroke	<1%	NR	Associated with seizures
Evening primrose (*Oenothera biennis*)	Ameliorates menopausal symptoms	NR	2%	Antiseizure effects (animals)	Possibly associated with seizures

(continued)

Table 2.2 Characteristics of Natural Products Used by People With Epilepsy in Countries With a Western-Based Type of Medical System[a] (*continued*)

Product	Main Current Medical Uses	Main Adverse Events & Interactions	Overall Estimated Extent of Use in PWEs[b]	Possible Effects in Epilepsy	Potential Risks for PWEs
Garlic	Antioxidant; prevents cardiovascular disease & cancer; immune stimulant	GI disturbance, dizziness; possible increase in INR, HTN, arrhythmia; possible influence on CYP3A4 & inhibitor of CYP2C9/19	10%	NR	NR
Ginger	Prevents cardiovascular disease & cancer; ameliorates GI symptoms; antioxidant; antiinflammatory	May increase risk of bleeding in warfarin users; possible inductor of CYP1A2 & 3A4	<1%	May have antiepileptic effects	NR
Ginkgo biloba	Cognitive enhancer; prevents cardiovascular disease; antioxidant	GI discomfort, anticoagulant; may inhibit CYP2B6 & induce CYP3A & 1A2, 2C19	16%	Leaves & stems may be anticonvulsive	Seeds may be toxic & proconvulsive; may increase metabolism of AED (PHT, VPA, PB)
Ginseng	Ameliorates anxiety, depression, concentration problems, DM, menopausal symptoms, & sexual dysfunction in men; stimulant	Possible hepatotoxicity & increased INR, lethargy	17%	May have anticonvulsive properties	May exacerbate seizures

Glucosamine	Antiarthritis; antiarthralgia	May increase INR in warfarin users	<1%	NR	NR
Glutamine	Enhances healing after injury, especially GI; promotes muscle building	NR	<1%	NR	NR
Goldenseal (*Hydrastis canadensis*)	Antiinflammatory; antimicrobial	Possible hypernatremia, HTN, edema; strong inhibitor of CYP2D6 & CYP3A4/5, CYP2E1	5%	NR	NR
Grapefruit juice	Prevents cardiovascular disease & cancer; antioxidant	Inhibits enteric CYP3A4, possibly increases risk of breast cancer	<1%	NR	Increases bioavailability of CBZ, BDZ
Grape seed	Prevents cardiovascular disease & cancer; antioxidant	Hypersensitivity, HA, dizziness, nausea; may inhibit CYP2E1	4%	NR	NR
Hops (*Humulus lupulus*)	Ameliorates anxiety, insomnia, & menopausal symptoms; antiinflammatory; antioxidant	Sedation; possibly inhibits CYP2C9, 1A1/2, 1B1	<1%	NR	Possibly exacerbates seizure
Kava kava (*Piper methysticum*)	Ameliorates depression, anxiety, & insomnia; induces local anesthesia	Possibly psychosis, choreoathetosis, hepatotoxicity, dermopathy, lymphopenia, GI disturbances, potential for addiction; inhibitor of CYP2E1, 1A2; induction of 1A1	4%	May benefit	Possibly exacerbate seizures

(continued)

Table 2.2 Characteristics of Natural Products Used by People With Epilepsy in Countries With a Western-Based Type of Medical System[a] (continued)

Product	Main Current Medical Uses	Main Adverse Events & Interactions	Overall Estimated Extent of Use in PWEs[b]	Possible Effects in Epilepsy	Potential Risks for PWEs
L-lysine	Precursor of carnitine; promotes protein building; anticancer; antiviral	NR	<1%	NR	NR
Licorice (liquorice or *Glycyrrhiza glabra*)	Expectorant; antiviral; antispasmodic; ameliorates gastric & duodenal ulcers & menopausal symptoms	In overdose: hypokalemia & increase in BP, decrease testosterone in men; may increase INR when taken with warfarin; possibly inhibits CYP3A4, 2B6, 2C9	2%	NR	NR
Marijuana (*Cannabis sativa*)	Antinociceptive; ameliorates glaucoma; antinausea; muscle relaxant; promotes bone health	Tachycardia, dry mouth, red eyes, euphoria, anxiety, psychosis, memory deficit; possibly induces CYP2E1		May benefit	May exacerbate seizures
Melatonin	Ameliorates insomnia, circadian rhythm abnormalities, depression, & anxiety	HA, nausea, somnolence	7%	May benefit	Associated with increased seizure frequency
Milk thistle	Ameliorates hepatotoxicity & DM; anticancer	Possible downregulation of CYP3A4, 2C9	<1%	NR	NR

Nettles (*Urtica dioica*)	Antinociceptive; antiarthritis; antioxidant; diuretic; ameliorates BHP	Uterine stimulant	<1%	NR	NR
Omega-3/fish oil	Cardioprotective; ameliorates depression, dementia, ADHD	Anticoagulant	<1%	May be beneficial (SUDEP)	NR
Parsley leaf	Diuretic; ameliorates constipation; promotes bone health	May increase INR when taken with warfarin; possibly downregulates P450; possibly stimulates uterine contractions	<1%	NR	NR
Saw palmetto (*Serenoa repens*)	Ameliorates UTI & BHP	GI disturbance, HA, decreased libido; inhibition of CYP3A4, 2D6, 2C9	2%	NR	NR
Skullcap (*Scutellaria*)	Sedative; antiepileptic; antihypnotic; antianxiolytic; anticancer	NR	<1%	May benefit	NR
Soy	Source of omega-3 & -6 fatty acids; ameliorates menopausal symptoms; prevents prostate cancer; promotes bone health	May increase risk of developing breast cancer; possibly inhibits CYP2A6, 1A1, 1B1, 3A4	8%	NR	NR

(continued)

Table 2.2 Characteristics of Natural Products Used by People With Epilepsy in Countries With a Western-Based Type of Medical System[a] *(continued)*

Product	Main Current Medical Uses	Main Adverse Events & Interactions	Overall Estimated Extent of Use in PWEs[b]	Possible Effects in Epilepsy	Potential Risks for PWEs
St. John's wort (*Hypericum perforatum*)	Ameliorates depression, pain, ADHD	Possibly hepatotoxicity, visual disturbances, paresthesia, myalgia, GI disturbances, sedation, photosensitivity; inducer of CYP3A4, 2E1, 2C19, P-glycoprotein; possible inhibition of CYP2C9/19, 2D6, 3A4, 1A2; avoid MAO inhibitors & SSRIs	13%	Possible benefit	Possibly associated with seizures
Valerian	Ameliorates anxiety, insomnia, & epilepsy; nociceptive	GI disturbance, drowsiness, HA; avoid barbiturates; possibly inhibits CYP2D6, 3A4	5%	May benefit	NR

[a]Only use of herbs and dietary supplements was studied.

[b]The overall extent of use was calculated by combining data from the publications that provided numerical data for the use of specific products. See Ekstein and Schachter (9) for details.

Abbreviations: ADHD, attention deficit/hyperactivity disorder; AED, antiepileptic drugs; BDZ, benzodiazepine; BHP, benign hypertrophy of prostate; BP, blood pressure; CBZ, carbamazepine; CHF, congestive heart failure; DHEA, dehydroepiandrosterone; DM, diabetes mellitus; GI, gastrointestinal; HA, headache; HTN, hypertension; INR, international normalized ratio; MAO, monoamine oxidase; NR, not reported; PB, phenobarbital; PHT, phenytoin; PWEs, people with epilepsy; SSRI, selective serotonin reuptake inhibitor; SUDEP, sudden unexplained death in epilepsy; UTI, urinary tract infection; VPA, valproic acid.

Reprinted with permission from Ekstein and Schachter (9).

Zizyphi Fructus); Paeoniae Radix; and Zheng Tai Instant Powder (a complex prescription of TCM used for tonic-clonic seizures) (Table 2.3) (16). Interestingly, scientific studies show that some of these herbal remedies protect brain cells and prevent seizures in animal models of epilepsy (16).

Practitioners of TCM often individualize their recommendations of herbal remedies to PWE, based on the TCM principles of holism and differentiation. This means that the same practitioner may recommend different herbal remedies to different PWE, even though they may have the same seizure type and frequency (14). As mentioned in the introduction, controlled trial evidence regarding recommendation of specific Asian herbal medicines, either alone or in combination, for PWE is lacking, and further research is needed.

Ayurveda

Ayurveda, the knowledge of life, is derived from 2 Sanskrit words: *ayu*, which means "life," and *veda*, which means "to know." Ayurveda originated as a traditional medical system in India nearly 8,000 years ago (17). Ayurvedic writings

Table 2.3   Herbal Remedies Used to Treat Convulsions in Asia

Herb	Note
Chai-Hu-Long-Ku-Mu-Li-Tan	Mixture of extracts from 13 herbal medicines
Gastrodia elata	
Uncaria rhynchophylla	
Menispermum dauricum	
Shitei-To	Mixture of extracts from 3 medicine herbs 1. Shitei: kaki calyx, calyx of *Diospyros kaki* L.f. 2. Shokyo: zingiberis rhizoma, rhizome of *Zingiber officinale* Roscoe 3. Choji: caryophylli flos, flower bud of *Syzygium aromaticum* L.
Qingyangshen (mixture of radish & pepper)	Contains alkaloid piperine
Kanbaku-Taiso-To	Mixture of 3 herbal drugs 1. Glycyrrhizae Radix 2. Tritici Semen 3. Zizyphi Fructus
Paeoniae Radix	
Zheng Tai Instant Powder	Complex prescription of traditional Chinese medicine used for tonic-clonic seizures

Reprinted with permission from Liow et al (16).

contain numerous references to symptoms consistent with epilepsy. Ayurvedic practitioners often encourage PWE to follow nutritional guidelines and to take herbal remedies, whether externally, internally, or topically. Examples of these remedies include Brahmi Rasayan, Brahmi Ghritham, Ashwagandha, old pure desi ghee, daily fresh juice of brahmi with honey, garlic juice in oil, and powdered root of wild asparagus with milk. Others include *Acacia arabica, Acorus calamus, Bacoppa monnieri, Clitorea turuatea, Celastrus panniculata, Convulvulus pluricaulis, Emblica officinalis,* Mukta pishti, *Whitania somnifera,* and Vaca brahmi yoga (16). Scientific studies have provided some evidence to suggest that these products have actions on brain cells that could be relevant to antiseizure treatments (16); however, further rigorous studies are needed before any of these treatments can be recommended to PWE.

Homeopathy

The term *homeopathy* comes from the Greek word *homoios*, which means "similar," and *pathos*, relating to suffering or disease. This medical system was first described by the Greek physician Hippocrates and then more formally codified by the German physician Samuel Hahnemann (1755–1843), who was particularly concerned with the severe toxicity of treatments used by doctors in his day. In homeopathy, "like should be cured with like," meaning that a homeopathic preparation used to treat symptoms incorporates a drug, often derived from plants or animal products, that itself causes similar symptoms when given to a healthy volunteer (18). Hahnemann proposed that this active ingredient should be repetitively diluted and vigorously shaken before it is taken by the patient (19). Based on homeopathic principles, specific treatments are recommended to a patient according to symptoms, or what is believed to be causing the symptoms, rather than on a specific diagnosis.

Homeopathic medicines are occasionally taken by PWE. Though the risks appear to be low because of the extreme dilution of the active ingredients, further research to determine their efficacy and safety is needed.

REGULATORY ASPECTS OF HERBAL MEDICINES IN THE UNITED STATES

People with epilepsy and their physicians should be aware of the differences in how the U.S. government oversees the production, animal and clinical testing, and labeling of pharmaceuticals and dietary supplements. Herbal remedies are regulated by the 1994 Dietary Supplement and Health Education Act, whereas the clinical development, manufacturing, and marketing of prescription drugs are regulated by the much more rigorous requirements of the Federal Food, Drug, and Cosmetic Act.

The Dietary Supplement and Health Education Act defines a dietary supplement as a product taken by mouth that contains a dietary ingredient intended to supplement the diet. The dietary ingredients in these products may include vitamins, minerals, herbs, or other botanicals; amino acids; and substances such as enzymes, organ tissues, glandulars, and metabolites (20). Manufacturers of herbal products are responsible for the truthfulness of the claims they make on product labels, for controlling the quality of their products, and verifying their safety. They cannot claim that their herbal product is effective against a specific disease or medical condition, such as epilepsy, but they may claim that it has some effect on a part of the body or its function as long as the claim is accompanied by the following words: "This statement has not been evaluated by the FDA. This product is not intended to diagnose, treat, cure, or prevent any disease."

No government agency, including the FDA, is required by law to independently review and verify the labeling claims and supporting evidence of herbal products or to independently verify the quality of herbal products and their safety. That is, the FDA does not "approve" dietary supplements based on evidence of safety and effectiveness. Similarly, no U.S. governmental agency is required to verify that the production of herbal products is consistent with the standards that are required for pharmaceutical products. Therefore, herbal products could potentially be contaminated with microorganisms, pesticides, or toxic metals, as was documented with some Ayurvedic herbal products sold commercially in the Boston area (21). Further, they could contain other herbs or drugs, and the potency and amount per pill/capsule may vary significantly from batch to batch.

To address this problem, in 2007, the FDA issued *Current Good Manufacturing Practice in Manufacturing, Packaging, Labeling, or Holding Operations for Dietary Supplements* (22), which, in time, may help to prevent significant variation in the amount of active ingredients in herbal/botanical products (23).

SAFETY ISSUES

Despite being natural, herbal remedies are not necessarily safe, and intoxication may be fatal. The long-term safety of most herbal remedies is unknown. The interactions between herbal remedies and AEDs, with few exceptions, are also unknown. Conry and Pearl (24) suggest that a number of these products, including St. John's wort, garlic, echinacea, pycnogel, milk thistle, American hellebore, mugwort, and pipsissewa, may potentially affect the serum concentrations of AEDs that are metabolized by the liver. In addition, as noted earlier, a number of herbal remedies have been reported to cause seizures or exacerbate seizure activity in PWE (16). Therefore, it is very important for PWE to openly and completely discuss their use of herbal remedies with their physicians. It is particularly concerning in this regard that many patients do not inform their physicians about their use of herbs and botanicals (11–12, 25–26).

CONCLUSION

Herbal remedies are widely used by PWE, but there is currently little evidence of their safety and effectiveness. People with epilepsy should be made aware of possible manufacturing issues as well as the potential for interactions with AEDs, side effects, and worsening seizures. Their use of herbal remedies should be discussed with physicians and monitored closely.

Despite these issues, based on a centuries-long history of use and emerging scientific evidence in the laboratory, some herbal remedies should be further tested using systematic and rigorous methods to explore their potential as new treatments for epilepsy.

REFERENCES

1. Kwan P, Brodie MJ. Early identification of refractory epilepsy. *N Engl J Med*. 2000; 342:314–319.
2. Kwan P, Arzimanoglou A, Berg AT, et al. Definition of drug resistant epilepsy: consensus proposal by the ad hoc Task Force of the ILAE Commission on Therapeutic Strategies. *Epilepsia*. 2009;51:1069–1077.
3. What Is Complementary and Alternative Medicine? National Center for Complementary and Alternative Medicine Web site. http://nccam.nih.gov/health/whatiscam/. Accessed April 18, 2012.
4. U.S. Food and Drug Administration Web site. http://www.fda/gov/AboutFDA/Centers-Offices/CDER/ucm090983.htm. Accessed April 18, 2012.
5. Li Q, Chen X, He L, Zhou D. Traditional Chinese medicine for epilepsy. *Cochrane Database Syst Rev*. 2009;8:CD006454.
6. Wells R, Phillips RS, Schachter SC, McCarthy EP. Complementary and alternative medicine use among U.S. adults with common neurological conditions. *J Neurol*. 2010;257:1822–1831.
7. Barnes PM, Bloom B, Nahin RL. Complementary and alternative medicine use among adults and children: United States, 2007. *Natl Health Stat Report*. 2008;10:1–23.
8. Nahin RL, Barnes PM, Stussman BJ, Bloom B. Costs of complementary and alternative medicine (CAM) and frequency of visits to CAM practitioners: United States, 2007. *Natl Health Stat Report*. 2009;18:1–14.
9. Ekstein D, Schachter SC. Natural products in epilepsy—the present situation and perspectives for the future. *Pharmaceuticals*. 2010;3:1426–1445.
10. LaFrance WC Jr, Kanner AM, Hermann B. Psychiatric comorbidities in epilepsy. *Int Rev Neurobiol*. 2008;83:347–383.
11. Peebles CT, McAuley JW, Roach J, Moore JL, Reeves AL. Alternative medicine use by patients with epilepsy. *Epilepsy Behav*. 2000;1:74–77.
12. Sirven JI, Drazkowski JF, Zimmerman RS, Bortz JJ, Shulman DL, Macleish M. Complementary/alternative medicine for epilepsy in Arizona. *Neurology*. 2003;61:576–577.
13. Pope NJ. Naturopathic medicine. In: Devinsky O, Schachter S, Pacia S, eds. *Complementary and Alternative Therapies for Epilepsy*. New York, NY: Demos Medical Publishing; 2005:165–176.
14. Wang S, Li Y. Traditional Chinese medicine. In: Devinsky O, Schachter S, Pacia S, eds. *Complementary and Alternative Therapies for Epilepsy*. New York, NY: Demos Medical Publishing; 2005:177–182.
15. Lai CW, Lai YH. History of epilepsy in Chinese traditional medicine. *Epilepsia*. 1991; 32:299–302.
16. Schachter SC, Acevedo C, Acevedo K, Lai CW, Diop AG. Complementary and alternative medical therapies. In: Engel J, Pedley TA, eds. *Epilepsy: A Comprehensive Textbook. 2nd ed*. Philadelphia, PA: Lippincott Williams and Wilkins; 2008:1407–1414.

17. Jain S. Ayurveda: the ancient Indian system of medicine. In: Devinsky O, Schachter S, Pacia S, eds. *Complementary and Alternative Therapies for Epilepsy.* New York, NY: Demos Medical Publishing; 2005:123–128.

18. Vickers A, Zollman C. ABC of complementary medicine: homoeopathy. *Br Med J.* 1999;319:1115–1118.

19. Taffler S. Homeopathy. In: Devinsky O, Schachter S, Pacia S, eds. *Complementary and Alternative Therapies for Epilepsy.* New York, NY: Demos Medical Publishing; 2005:157–164.

20. U.S. Food and Drug Administration Web site. http://www.cfsan.fda.gov/~dms/ds-oview.html. Accessed February 25, 2011.

21. Saper RB, Kales SN, Paquin J, et al. Heavy metal content of ayurvedic herbal medicine products. *JAMA.* 2004;292:2868–2873.

22. Current Good Manufacturing Practice in Manufacturing, Packaging, Labeling, or Holding Operations for Dietary Supplements. U.S. Food and Drug Administration Web site. http://www.fda.gov/ohrms/dockets/98fr/cf0441.pdf. Accessed April 18, 2012.

23. Garrard J, Harms S, Eberly LE, Matiak A. Variations in product choices of frequently purchased herbs: caveat emptor. *Arch Intern Med.* 2003;163:2290–2295.

24. Conry JA, Pearl PL. Herbal therapy in epilepsy. In: Devinsky O, Schachter S, Pacia S, eds. *Complementary and Alternative Therapies for Epilepsy.* New York, NY: Demos Medical Publishing; 2005:129–142.

25. Gidal BE, Sheth RD, Bainbridge J, et al. Alternative medicine (AM) use in epilepsy: results of a national, multicenter survey. *Epilepsia.* 1999;40(suppl 7):107–108.

26. Liow K, Ablah E, Nguyen JC, Sadler T, Wolfe D, Tran KD. Pattern and frequency of use of complementary and alternative medicine among patients with epilepsy in the midwestern United States. *Epilepsy Behav.* 2007;10:576–582.

3

Nutrition

Nutrition is a foundation for health. Mainstream and alternative approaches to health care recognize the importance of diet. The scientific study of nutrition trails far behind molecular and pharmaceutical research. Identifying, preventing, and treating nutritional deficiencies such as scurvy and rickets helped determine the course of how mainstream and alternative medical efforts view nutrition. Supplementation became a key principle. The original doctrine of replacing deficiencies in nutrition has evolved into the philosophy "some is good, more is better"—but how much is good? Of equal merit, how much is better, and when is it better? Is more ever worse? Current American Dietetic Association minimal dietary requirements for vitamins and minerals reflect informed opinion as well as fact. Everything in moderation; excess can be injurious. Too much vitamin B_6 (>250 mg/d for long periods) can damage sensory nerves. Too much vitamin D during pregnancy may cause congenital malformations. Yet deficiencies remain despite knowledge and availability. Rickets was first described in 1645. Seventeenth-century folklore held that cod liver oil (rich in vitamin D) could prevent rickets. This claim was endorsed by doctors in the early 1800s and confirmed in the early 1900s. However, vitamin D deficiency still plagues our society as osteoporosis.

Many nutritional disorders result from the dramatic dietary changes that accompany civilization. Nutritional experts still hotly debate the "best diet" for health. Some hold carbohydrates to be the main culprits in promoting disease, while others advocate the role of high-fat, high-calorie, high-meat, animal-based (meat, fish, and dairy) or micronutrient-based diets as unhealthy. Our genes and bodies primarily evolved to consume a hunter-gatherer diet. Our lack of mental and physical adaptations to our diet has led to the obesity epidemic from excess carbohydrate consumption, often compounded by high fat consumption. Similarly, excess salt consumption contributes to hypertension in susceptible populations. However, some adaptations do occur. During the past 7,000 years, many pastoral human groups passed on a mutation in chromosome 2 that permits lactase production after weaning. This novel change provided these groups with an additional food resource since lactose intolerance is the normal mammalian condition after breastfeeding. Other adaptations help in some settings but hurt us in others. People of Mediterranean heritage may have a glucose-6-phosphate dehydrogenase deficiency that provides some protection against malaria but makes them vulnerable to serious anemia if they are ill, eat broad (fava) beans, or are exposed to certain chemicals. It is possible that genetic alterations in ion channel and neurotransmitter receptor proteins that contribute to epilepsy risk evolved as adaptations to certain environmental conditions, including nutrition.

Modern life has also added substances to foods that our bodies were not exposed to during millions of years of hominid evolution. The adverse health consequences of dietary contaminants and additives remain poorly defined. In contrast to the role of asbestos in causing mesothelioma, the role of dietary chemicals in cancer, although many are suspected (e.g., sodium nitrite, butylated hydroxyanisole), is difficult to prove. Extrapolations from animal studies using doses that far exceed known human exposure are of uncertain significance (1).

It is critical to distinguish association and causation. High urinary concentrations of pesticides (organophosphates) were found in the urine of children with attention deficit/hyperactivity disorder (2). This study showed an association, not causation. Other contaminants such as mercury are very elevated in tuna, swordfish, and other large predatory fish. Although mercury poisoning does not cause seizures, it can cause neurologic and psychiatric symptoms. In susceptible individuals, mercury toxicity may lower the seizure threshold. The role of food additives (e.g., aspartame) in modifying seizure threshold is discussed below. For seizures and epilepsy, we lack data on the effect of foods and diets, nutritional deficiencies, and supplements—with some notable exceptions.

Albert Schweitzer (1875–1965), medical missionary and Nobel laureate, worked more than 4 decades in Gabon, caring for over 150,000 and operating on more than 5,000 people. At first, cancer and appendicitis were exceedingly rare. However, as the native diet and lifestyle were westernized, these disorders became more common. Similarly, as the diet of remote Eskimo populations in coastal Labrador westernized, cancer rates increased (3). Unlike some disorders, epilepsy commonly affects sub-Saharan Africans because of infections such as HIV, malaria, and neurocysticercosis. If a lower incidence of epilepsy resulted from a non-Western lifestyle, it would require detailed data on epilepsy etiology, which is often lacking in areas in the developing world owing to lack of access to medical care and limited diagnostic testing.

Epidemiologic studies link certain diseases with nutrition, food supplements, pesticides, and lifestyle factors. In most cases, the data show only an association. For epilepsy, we often lack even epidemiologic data showing associations. Apart from the modified Atkins and ketogenic diets (see below), no nutritional programs, foods, or supplements definitely help control seizures. Similarly, we do not know if any nutritional programs, foods, or supplements definitely increase seizure activity, although many drugs can do this. Since low carbohydrate diets can reduce seizures, do high carbohydrate diets increase seizure activity? It does not seem like this is a common occurrence, but we do not know.

The American Dietetic Association position paper on functional foods reviews the evidence that nutritional supplements modify disease risk (4). The FDA authorized 7 health claims under the Nutrition Labeling and Education Act. Of these claims, none relate to epilepsy. Most concern a decreased risk of cardiovascular disease (e.g., whole oat, psyllium seed husk, barley fiber, soy protein, plant stanol, and sterol esters). Less convincing studies support a variety of other dietary components in reducing cardiovascular risk (e.g., almonds and hazelnuts; vitamins B_6, B_{12}, and folic acid; ω-3 fatty acids, monosaturated fats from olive oil) as well as cancer risk (e.g., tomatoes: prostate, ovarian, gastric, and pancreatic cancer; green tea: breast and prostate cancer; calcium: colon cancer) (4). There has been little systematic study of nutritional supplements in epilepsy.

The traditional "balanced" diet recommended by the American Dietetic Association consists of a mixture high in carbohydrates, moderate in protein, and low in fats. Many researchers criticize this food pyramid model that has been the framework for a healthy diet for nearly 30 years. Studies on the Atkins diet (high protein, low carbohydrate) support its value for weight loss, but there is no evidence relating its effects on seizures or long-term safety (5). A modified Atkins diet with very limited carbohydrate consumption (see below) and the ketogenic diet, one that is high in fat, low in protein, and extremely low in carbohydrates, can help control seizures in some patients (see below). Fasting rarely provokes seizures and actually may reduce seizure frequency by putting the body in a state of ketosis (6–7). Hypoglycemia, a drop in blood sugar below the normal limits, could possibly provoke seizure activity, although it is not common unless the decline is very severe (8–9).

Very rarely, specific metabolic deficiencies, such as pyridoxine (vitamin B_6) deficiency, cause epilepsy. Such seizures usually occur very early in life and are exquisitely responsive to pyridoxine replacement. Tissues with high energy consumption, such as the brain, heart, and muscle, depend on the mitochondria to produce energy in the cell. These tissues are sensitive to mitochondrial dysfunction. Certain diets (e.g., more frequent meals/snacks with some glucose and electrolytes) and supplements (e.g., antioxidants) help some patients with mitochondrial disorders and may improve seizure control (10–11). However, scant evidence links dietary changes or supplements with improved seizure control in these patients, and there are no data that "mito diets or supplements" improve seizure control in patients with normal mitochondria.

Apart from the modified Atkins and ketogenic diets, no solid evidence links dietary changes with changes in seizure activity. Individual patients report that certain foods (e.g., high sugar content, nitrite-containing hot dogs) or additives (e.g., aspartame) can trigger seizures. Scientific studies do not confirm these associations (12–13). Similarly, some people with epilepsy take antioxidants and free radical scavengers such as ω-3 fatty acids and vitamin E (14–16). Although these compounds may reduce cancer risk and slow the progression of neurodegenerative disorders such as Alzheimer and Parkinson disease (17–18), no evidence supports the claim that antioxidants reduce seizure activity or reduce the consequences of chronic epilepsy, such as impaired short-term memory. Many physicians and lay people believe that the benefits of these nutritional/vitamin supplements outweigh the risks. However, some studies have linked vitamin E supplementation with an increased risk of some cancers. Until more data are available, the true risk-benefit ratio remains uncertain.

The more we understand the biochemical pathways and molecular processes that cause seizures, the more we may understand the pathways and processes behind healthy neuronal function. Medical research focuses on basic mechanisms and translational strategies centered on drug and device development. We must also study how diet affects epilepsy and how epilepsy impacts metabolism and nutritional needs. Amino acids, vitamins, and minerals are essential components of daily metabolism, and their concentrations may affect seizure threshold or, vice versa, epilepsy may affect their concentrations. Studies are beginning to look at both the preventative and therapeutic roles nutrition can play in the treatment of epilepsy. The efficacy of low-carbohydrate diets has fueled interest in novel "dietary drugs" such as 2-deoxyglucose (addressed later in this chapter). Because of the broad spectrum of causes for epilepsy, treatments must be chosen carefully, and the findings of one particular study may not apply to all people with epilepsy.

THE KETOGENIC DIET

In the 1920s, a diet consisting mostly of fats dramatically reduced the frequency of seizures in many children. The diet was named the "ketogenic diet" because it caused ketosis, a state where the body produces ketone bodies by metabolizing fat and protein. The 3 major ketone bodies are acetone, acetoacetic acid, and β-hydroxybutyric acid, although the latter is actually a carboxylic acid. After phenytoin was introduced in 1938, the ketogenic diet was rarely used. The diet's value has been reaffirmed, and its popularity has grown during the past 25 years (19–21). We remain uncertain as to how diet controls seizures. Leading theories include changes in pH; increased energy production; resistance to metabolic stress, amino acids, and ketones (22). A recent consensus statement and review provides an excellent clinical overview (23).

The diet has limitations, such as one's ability to abide by the restrictions and social-emotional dysfunction, and side effects, such as kidney stones, growth retardation, constipation, and metabolic disorders. The modified Atkins and low glycemic (South Beach) diets also restrict carbohydrates but allow more protein, thereby increasing tolerability and compliance while decreasing side effects. These less restrictive alternatives appear to be equally effective in some patients (24).

The ketogenic diet can improve seizure control in many age and seizure groups. The greatest experience and success are with children between ages 18 months and 6 years whose seizures cannot be controlled by AEDs. This is especially true for children with Lennox-Gastaut, Doose, Dravet, Rett, and infantile spasm syndromes who have atonic, tonic, and myoclonic seizures (25–26).

However, controlled studies show similar efficacy in children with symptomatic generalized and symptomatic focal epilepsies (20). After the age of 3 years, children have usually been exposed to foods that they are unwilling to part with. Therefore, older children and adults who can choose their food must be highly motivated to stay on the ketogenic diet. In sensitive patients, consuming even small amounts of forbidden carbohydrates, or even proteins, can worsen seizure control. Thus, many parents are hesitant to try the ketogenic diet because their child loves carbohydrates or is a finicky eater. For children with severe epilepsy, however, the potential benefits of a 1- to 3-month trial outweigh the risks.

Contraindications to using the ketogenic diet include metabolic disorders of fatty acid transport or oxidation, primary carnitine deficiency, pyruvate decarboxylase deficiency, and porphyria. Relative contraindications include patients who have poor baseline nutrition, noncompliant parents or caregivers, or those with a seizure focus with concordant imaging and video electroencephalographic (EEG) data which can benefit from epilepsy surgery (24).

Although this diet can be used successfully in adults, patients often find the modified Atkins or low glycemic diets more tolerable. Infants who are fed only formula or children who are fed only with a gastrostomy tube can be easily put on the ketogenic diet. KetoCal is a commercially available ketogenic powder that can be dissolved in warm water (113°F to 122°F) and provides a 4:1 ratio of fats to other nutrients.

The ketogenic diet is most often used in epilepsy centers for children with uncontrolled seizures. A knowledgeable dietician and physician should supervise the diet. Individual modifications are often needed to make it more effective or tolerable. Before starting the diet, a baseline evaluation and blood work should be obtained (Table 3.1).

Table 3.1   Evaluation Before Starting Ketogenic Diet

Counseling	Discuss expectations and plans for implementation
	Review potential obstacles and ways to enhance compliance
	Identify potential hidden sources of carbohydrates (e.g., medication elixirs)
	Reliable educational materials (books, videos, Web, discussion groups)
Nutritional evaluation	Measure height and weight
	Consultation with nutritionist 1. Review history for preferences, allergies, and intolerances 2. Determine calories, dietary composition (e.g., ratio), and fluid 3. Determine supplementation
	Select type of ketogenic diet: classic or MCT, modified Atkins, or low glycemic

(*continued*)

Table 3.1   Evaluation Before Starting Ketogenic Diet (*continued*)

Laboratory evaluation	Complete blood cell count
	Serum 1. Electrolytes 2. Bicarbonate 3. Renal and liver functions 4. Total protein and albumin 5. Essential minerals: zinc, selenium, magnesium, phosphorus 6. Lipid profile (fasting) 7. Acylcarnitine profile (intermediates in fatty acid oxidation) 8. Amino acids 9. Trough antiepileptic drug levels
Urine	Urinalysis
	Calcium, creatinine
	Organic acids

Abbreviation: MCT, mixed chain triglyceride.

The classical "Johns Hopkins" approach initiated the diet in the hospital with a 24- to 48-hour fast with limited fluids. This starvation period lowered the child's blood sugar, which could result in pallor, diaphoresis, tremulousness, irritability, confusion, decreased level of responsiveness, vomiting, or even seizures. In such cases, the child requires sugar or other carbohydrate supplementation to prevent more serious side effects. Fluid restriction can cause dehydration. After starvation, ketogenic food is gradually introduced. There is no proof that either fluid or calorie restriction when beginning the diet is beneficial (27).

Many epilepsy centers initiate the diet outside of the hospital without starvation or fluid restrictions. This more gradual outpatient regimen has fewer side effects, less physical and emotional stress, and reduced costs. Controlled studies demonstrate that when compared with the rapid starvation initiation, the gradual approach has equal efficacy and fewer side effects (28). Problems during starvation lead some patients and parents to give up on the diet before it has a chance to demonstrate its benefit. The diet can be monitored with urine ketones measured at home with an indicator strip. Urine ketones show that the diet has achieved its metabolic goal of ketosis; higher ketone levels correlate with improved seizure control in many children.

The ketogenic diet consists primarily of foods high in fat, with most of the remaining calories made up of proteins. With the commonly used 3:1 or 4:1 ratios of fats to carbohydrates and protein, 70% to 90% of the foods are fats, and 10% to 30% are carbohydrates and protein. Studies have shown that the 4:1 ratio provides better control of seizures, but many patients can be transitioned from a 4:1 to a 3:1 ratio with improved dietary tolerability and fewer gastrointestinal (GI) side effects (29). The daily diet often consists of 35 to 45 calories (145–188 Joules) per pound (75–100 calories/kg (315–420 J/kg)) and 0.5 to 1.0 g of protein per pound (1–2 g/kg) of body weight. Examples of high-fat foods include mayonnaise, butter, and heavy cream. The foods must be carefully measured and weighed. Only small portions of cheese, meat, fish, or poultry are allowed each day. Fruit is allowed in small amounts.

Mixed chain triglycerides (MCTs) (Liquigen, SHS, Liverpool UK, Medical Supplement) are an alternative fat source; MCT is a clear, light-colored flavorless oil but can also be a coconut oil or an emulsion. The use of MCT oil allows for more nonfat foods. The laxative properties of MCT help counteract the constipating effects of the diet. Mixed chain triglycerides are sometimes used to supplement the traditional ketogenic diet to produce ketosis and relieve constipation. Mixed chain triglyceride oil should be introduced gradually to avoid stomach cramps. The traditional MCT oil diet derived 60% of the caloric intake from MCT. A modified form, with fewer GI side effects, derives 30% to 50% of calories from MCT and 10% to 30% from long-chain fat (27). The MCT diet incorporates MCT oil into every meal. If GI tolerability is a problem, more frequent, smaller meals may help. A recent randomized trial compared the classical and MCT forms of the ketogenic diet and found comparable efficacy and tolerability (21). Notably, the small but significant differences were decreased energy (at 3 months) and more vomiting (at 12 months) in the classical group.

Because sugar is prohibited in the diet, parents must be vigilant about their children's medications, cough syrups, vitamins, toothpaste, and any other nonfoods or foods that may contain sugar. Small amounts of sugar can reverse the effects of the diet and cause a seizure. All adults who may be with the child in the parents' absence must be informed of the dietary restrictions.

Most centers recommend trying the diet for at least 2 to 3 months to determine if it is effective. However, one study found that 75% of those who eventually benefit from the diet responded within 2 weeks (27). Thus, shorter trials may be informative. If the diet is well tolerated and effective, the doctor usually continues it for 1 to 3 years. In patients with more than 90% seizure reduction in whom the diet is well tolerated, it may be continued for more than 5 years. Afterward, carbohydrates are gradually increased, typically over 2 to 6 months. Suddenly stopping the diet may cause a temporary increase in seizures. After the diet is discontinued, some children remain seizure-free without medications. However, seizures may recur, in which case they may be well controlled with medications that were ineffective before the diet. A patient who was seizure-free on a lower ratio of fats to protein and carbohydrates (e.g., 2.75:1), but whose seizures recurred when the diet was discontinued, may be helped by continuing the diet at a reduced ratio or trying the modified Atkins or low glycemic diets (see below).

If a child takes high doses of several AEDs, tapering of one drug is started around the time the diet is started. If ketosis is maintained and seizure control improves, a further reduction in medications is often possible. Occasionally, all medications can be tapered and stopped. The carbohydrate content of medications, often significant in liquid formulations, must be considered in calculating total carbohydrates.

The success of the ketogenic diet varies. One recent randomized study found that 38% in the diet group had greater than 50% seizure reduction compared with 6% among controls; 7% in the diet group had a greater than 90% seizure reduction compared with no controls (not significant) (20). Prior studies found higher success rates: after 1 year, 25% of patients experienced at least a 90% reduction in seizures, another 20% had a 50% to 90% reduction, and the remainder either did not tolerate or did not benefit from the diet (19). One meta-analysis found that 77% of patients discontinued the diet because of limited benefits (<50% seizure reduction, 47% of patients), dietary restrictions (16.5%), or intercurrent illness or diet side effects (13%) (30).

The long-term effects of a high-fat diet, even if it is only used for several years, are unknown. Brain development and intellectual/social functions can improve with better seizure control and reduced AED burden. Many parents worry about the effects of increased dietary fat. Although the ketogenic diet raises "bad" lipids (very-low-density lipoprotein and low-density lipoprotein) and can lower "good" lipids (high-density lipoprotein), there is no evidence of increased atherosclerosis in children or adolescents. However, this has not been adequately studied with long-term use of the diet. Weight gain is not usually a problem because caloric intake is carefully supervised.

An initial starvation period can cause dangerous hypoglycemia requiring urgent treatment. Other potential problems include a deficiency of the vitamins B, C, and D; calcium; folate; and iron. Therefore, these nutrients must be supplemented (Table 3.2). The ketogenic diet often slows a child's growth in height and weight, but this is often made up for, at least partially, when the diet is stopped. There is a risk of kidney stones, which can be reduced by adequate fluid intake and potassium citrate (Polycitra-K) (31). Although acetazolamide, topiramate,

Table 3.2 Supplements Recommended for Children on the Ketogenic Diet

Required	Multivitamin with trace minerals (carbohydrate free)
	Calcium
	Vitamin D
Optional	Potassium citate (Polycitra-K): prevent renal stones
	Selenium (20 ng/d)
	Zinc (50 mg/d)
	Phosphorus
	Carnitine
	MCT oil: increase ketosis or reduce constipation
	Laxatives (MiraLAX, mineral oil, glycerin suppository)

Abbreviation: MCT, mixed chain triglyceride.

Table 3.3 Follow-up Evaluations on Ketogenic Diet

Frequency	Every 3 months for first year: may be less frequent after; consider more frequent visits in children <1 year old
Nutritional assessment	Chart height, weight, and growth curve
	Assess tolerability and compliance of diet
	Review and modify as needed: calories, food content, ratio, fluids
	Review vitamin and other supplements
Neurological assessment	Review efficacy and tolerability of diet
	Consider reduction in antiepileptic drugs
Laboratory evaluation	Complete blood cell count
	Serum
	1. Electrolytes
	2. Bicarbonate
	3. Renal and liver functions
	4. Total protein and albumin
	5. Lipid profile (fasting)
	6. Acylcarnitine profile
	7. Amino acids
	8. Trough antiepileptic drug levels
Urine testing	Urinalysis
	Calcium, creatinine
Optional test	Serum beta-hydroxybutyrate (especially when urine ketones do not correlate with seizure control)
	Essential minerals: zinc, selenium, magnesium, phosphorus
	Urine specific gravity: ensure hydration (<1.105)
	DEXA (bone density): after 1 year
	Renal ultrasound

Abbreviation: DEXA, dual energy X-ray absorptiometry.

and zonisamide also predispose to kidney stones, with proper hydration on the diet, these drugs can still be used. Other complications include constipation and an increased risk of bone fractures.

The Internet provides a rich source of medical and parental wisdom (e.g., epilepsy.com, charliefoundation.org, matthewsfriends.org), but patients should be wary of opinions from one individual or an unknown website. The Internet has everything from recipes and personal observations to supportive chat rooms. There are several informative books: *Ketogenic Diets: Treatment for Epilepsies and Other Disorders* (by Eric Kossof and others, 2011), *Keto Kid: Helping Your Child Succeed on the Ketogenic Diet* (by Deborah Snider, 2006), and *The Keto Cookbook: Innovative Delicious Meals for Staying on the Ketogenic Diet* (Demos Health, NY, 2011).

THE MODIFIED ATKINS AND LOW GLYCEMIC DIETS

The modified Atkins and low glycemic diets are alternatives to the ketogenic diet. There are not yet controlled studies that compare either of these diets with the ketogenic diet, but the diets appear to have similar efficacy with fewer complications and problems (27). Unlike the ketogenic diet, the modified Atkins and low glycemic diets have no restrictions on protein intake, total calories, or fluids. They do not require hospitalization, initial fast, or careful calculations and weighing of food. As with the ketogenic diet, both diets produce ketosis; therefore, it can be helpful to monitor urinary ketones with indicator strips. These more liberal diets are easier for people to comply with. The use of the Atkins and low glycemic diets by millions of people for weight loss and diabetes provides a wealth of information.

Compared with the ketogenic diet, a major advantage of the modified Atkins/ low glycemic diets is more diverse foods and greater adherence. The unrestricted protein intake may be healthier for growing children. However, excess protein consumption (>50% of calories) can cause toxicity, including vomiting and decreased appetite. The modified Atkins and low glycemic diets do not require high fat content, which is an integral part of the ketogenic diet and can accelerate atherosclerosis. However, the modified Atkins diet does encourage fat intake. In some cases, seizure control improves when the percentage of fat calories increases. A doctor and a dietician should ideally supervise these diets. Weight and height should be monitored, as well as cholesterol and triglyceride levels, owing to increased fat intake. Possible side effects include weight loss (which may be good or bad!) and, for the modified Atkins diet, elevated cholesterol levels. It is uncertain if the risk of kidney stones is increased.

The modified Atkins diet encourages more fat intake and less carbohydrate intake (10–20 g/d) than the original Atkins diet. The low glycemic diet is less restrictive of total carbohydrates (approximately 40–60 g/d) but limits them to those with a low glycemic index. This index measures how quickly a carbohydrate increases the blood sugar level in comparison to table sugar. Carbohydrates with a low glycemic index cause a slower and more gradual increase in blood sugar; those with a high glycemic index cause a more rapid increase in blood sugar. The low glycemic diet encourages carbohydrates with a low glycemic index (<50–55 on the index; see glycemicindex.com or diabetes.ca/Section_About/glycemic. asp). These carbohydrates also have health benefits by reducing cholesterol and appetite and by lowering the risk of diabetes and heart disease. The South Beach diet incorporates low glycemic carbohydrates into the diet. However, in contrast to the Atkins diet, which allows all types of fats, the South Beach diet encourages the healthier, unsaturated fats.

VITAMINS, AMINO ACIDS, MINERALS, AND OTHER NUTRITIONAL SUPPLEMENTS

No scientific data support the claim that vitamins, amino acids, and other nutritional supplements can improve seizure control in the general population with epilepsy. Rarely, nutritional deficiencies of magnesium; calcium, and vitamin B_6 (a very rare cause of seizures in newborns) can cause seizures that improve with supplementation. Hypoglycemia resulting from insulin overdose or an insulin-secreting tumor can also cause seizures that respond to glucose. In contrast to these-well established but very uncommon deficiency states, there are unconfirmed claims and reports that supplementation with magnesium; calcium; vitamin E; vitamin B_{12}; melatonin; omega fatty acids; and the amino acids L-taurine, L-tyrosine, and dimethylglycine can reduce seizures in some patients. These claims are based on very limited human data from studies that are usually not controlled or blinded and also are comprised of very small patient numbers. While some claims are supported by animal models of epilepsy, less than 1% of compounds that show anticonvulsant properties for animals are considered candidates for human treatment. The primary reason for this discrepancy is concern regarding the effectiveness and safety of the drug in humans.

There is an enormous gap between anecdotal observation in humans and scientific study in animals in the context of safe and effective therapy. For example, many scientific studies show that omega fatty acids can reduce seizures in animal models (32). However, a randomized trial of polyunsaturated fatty acids in people with epilepsy showed no benefits (33). In this case, neither finding an antiepileptic effect in an animal model nor expecting a benefit based on the nutrient's role in brain physiology translated into a beneficial effect on seizure control. However, the study does not fully exclude a possible beneficial effect since a potential benefit—or harm—may be detectable only after a longer time or higher dose. However, the negative randomized study suggests that if such a benefit or harm occurs, it is probably a small effect. We need more blinded, controlled, and randomized studies with sufficiently powered samples (large patient populations) to answer these questions.

ANTIOXIDANTS AND VITAMINS

Antioxidants remove free radical intermediates and inhibit oxidation reactions. Oxidation reactions transfer electrons from one substance to an oxidizing agent and can produce free radicals. Free radicals are created as by-products of metabolism that can initiate chain reactions that disrupt/injure the cell membrane, mitochondria, and other cellular components. The brain is especially vulnerable to oxidative injury because of its high metabolic rate and elevated levels of polyunsaturated lipids, the target of lipid peroxidation. Antioxidants terminate these chain reactions by receiving the electrons from free radical intermediates and inhibit other oxidation reactions. Common antioxidants are often reducing agents, such as vitamin C, vitamin E (α-tocopherol), other tocopherols, thiols (organosulfur compounds or mercaptans), or polyphenols. Antioxidant compounds and foods in which they are found are summarized in Table 3.4.

Table 3.4   Foods Containing Antioxidants

Antioxidant Compounds	Foods Containing High Levels of Antioxidants
Vitamin C (ascorbic acid)	Fruits: citrus, berries
	Vegetables: broccoli, red pepper
	Antioxidant level is higher when fruits and vegetables are fresh and uncooked
Vitamin E (tocopherols, tocotrienols)	Vegetables oils
	Almonds
	Hazelnuts
	Avocados
	Eggs
	Milk
	Leafy green vegetables
	Wheat germ
	Whole grains
Phytolexin (e.g. resveratol)	Red wine
	Red grape skins
	Peanuts
	Blueberries
Flavonoids	White and green tea
	Fruit: citrus, berries
	Red onions
	Dark chocolate
	Red wine
Cartenoids (lycopene, carotenes, lutein)	Fruit: apricot, oranges
	Vegetables: carrots, tomatoes
	eggs

A dangerous myth is that if something is necessary for health, like anti-oxidants, more of it will make you healthier. Too much of a good thing is bad. Antioxidants that are strong reducing acids bind dietary minerals such as iron and zinc and prevent their absorption from the gut (34). Antioxidant supplements are associated with higher rates of cancer and mortality in large studies and meta-analyses (35–37). It is unclear if these findings extend to the general population, for many groups consisted of primarily elderly subjects, but the studies strongly remind us of the ancient maxim: everything in moderation.

Free radicals could hypothetically lower the seizure threshold through several mechanisms, including inactivation of glutamine synthase and glutamate decarboxylase, as well as effects on mitochondrial function. Glutamine synthase metabolizes glutamate, and its inhibition can increase glutamate levels. Glutamate decarboxylase converts glutamate to γ-aminobutyric acid (GABA), and its inhibition can depress GABA levels and elevate glutamate levels (38). Oxidative stress to mitochondrial systems can affect neuronal excitability and increase seizure susceptibility (39). Thus, mitochondrial oxidative injury may result from seizures and also contribute to epileptogenesis (39). Notably, ketones produced in the ketogenic diet reduce oxidative stress (40).

Although some data suggest that antioxidant levels are depressed in people with epilepsy, the largest and most rigorous study to date found no reduction in seizures with antioxidant therapy (41). People with epilepsy have increased oxidative stress when compared with nonepileptic controls (38). Children with epilepsy who are on AEDs have lower α-tocopherol (a form of vitamin E) levels than controls (15, 42). A double-blind placebo-controlled study on 24 patients with medically refractory epilepsy found that patients treated with 400 IU/d of vitamin E in addition to their regular medication experienced a significant reduction in seizures. The placebo group experienced no change in their seizure activity (14–15). One study in patients with refractory epilepsy found that an antioxidant supplement reduced seizure frequency (43). A randomized, double-blind, placebo-controlled study found no reduction in seizures in people with epilepsy treated with α-tocopherol for 3 months (41). It is possible that higher doses or longer duration of therapy may be needed to see an effect.

Vitamin B_6 (pyridoxine, primarily, but there are 6 other forms including pyridoxal and pyridoxamine) plays an essential role in synthesizing numerous neurotransmitters, balancing sodium and potassium levels, and lowering levels of homocysteine (a nonprotein amino acid; high levels correlate with cardiovascular disease). Vitamin B_6 is primarily obtained from meat and dairy products. It is a component of multiple enzymes involved in amino acid assembly into proteins and hormones and is also involved in protein catabolism. Several decarboxylase enzymes also require vitamin B_6. For example, glutamate decarboxylase uses the vitamin to convert glutamate into GABA. Deficiency of vitamin B_6 can reduce activity of glutamate decarboxylase, which may increase seizure activity, owing to decreased GABA levels. A vitamin B_6 deficiency, which we will later discuss, that causes seizures in newborns is well documented but extremely rare. The role of routine vitamin B_6 supplementation in children or adults with epilepsy is not established, and there are no controlled studies to support it. Doses of 50 to 150 mg of vitamin B_6 are often used to help counteract the behavioral side effects of levetiracetam, although controlled studies are lacking (44). Excessive amounts of vitamin B_6 can damage sensory nerves, resulting in numbness in the hands and feet (45–46). More research is needed to determine the extent to which vitamin B_6 can provide therapeutic efficacy in seizure control.

Very rare genetic vitamin B_6 dependency disorders can cause severe neonatal seizures and are associated with mental disability. These disorders require lifelong supplementation of B_6 (47). Four genetic conditions are known to cause vitamin B_6-dependent seizures. Reduced synthesis or availability of pyridoxal-5'-phosphate, pyridoxine cofactor, causes pyridoxine-phosphate oxidase deficiency or infantile hypophosphatasia. Increased use or inactivation of this molecule results in pyridoxine-dependent epilepsy or hyperprolinemia (type II). These disorders usually present with treatment-resistant seizures, mainly myoclonic, in the neonatal period. The EEG can be normal but often shows a slowing or a burst suppression pattern or hypsarrythmia. The disorders can be diagnosed by specific biomarkers and confirmed with molecular genetic studies (48). When patients are taken off vitamin B_6 therapy, seizures return immediately. Some researchers postulate that the developmental outcome of the child is dependent upon the dosage of vitamin B_6.

AMINO ACIDS

Amino acids are the building blocks for proteins. The body relies upon approximately 23 different amino acids, 8 of which are essential and are obtained only through the diet since the body cannot synthesize them. Amino acids occur naturally in most foods and are found in high concentrations in animal-based foods such as meat, fish, and eggs. Epilepsy can be simplified as an imbalance of brain electrical activity, resulting from too much excitation or too little inhibition. Concentrations of the excitatory neurotransmitters (mainly amino acids glutamate and aspartate) increase in the brain during and shortly after a seizure (49). Inhibitory amino acid neurotransmitters or their derivatives (GABA, glycine, and taurine) reduce electrical excitability. In theory, seizures could be prevented by supplementing the diet with inhibitory amino acid neurotransmitters or by restricting dietary input of excitatory amino acid neurotransmitters. However, several aspects of physiology make this simple goal problematic: (a) amino acids are charged and do not readily cross the blood-brain barrier but require specific carriers to ferry them across; (b) the body can synthesize the major excitatory and inhibitory amino acids and the neurotransmitters derived from them (except for tryptophan), so brain concentrations may not vary with dietary intake even if there were no blood-brain barrier; and (c) there are strong homeostatic mechanisms that maintain a balance between excitation and inhibition. Thus, oversupply of one amino acid can lead to increased excretion or increased synthesis of an opposing amino acid or both. There is no evidence that supplementing or restricting dietary amino acids affects seizure activity in humans.

γ-AMINOBUTYRIC ACID

The amino acid derivative GABA is the main inhibitory neurotransmitter in the nervous system. γ-Aminobutyric acid is chemically an amino acid but is usually not referred to as one since it is not incorporated into proteins and is not an alpha amino acid. γ-Aminobutyric acid synthesis starts with the conversion of glucose to glutamate through several enzymatic steps including glutamate dehydrogenase. Glutamate, the nervous system's main excitatory neurotransmitter, is converted to GABA by glutamate decarboxylase. Overactivity of glutamate dehydrogenase and/or underactivity of glutamate decarboxylase increases the ratio of glutamate to GABA, increasing brain excitability and lowering the seizure threshold.

Many antiepileptic drugs (AEDs) work by influencing GABA activity (50). Vigabatrin (Sabril) blocks the enzyme GABA transaminase, which metabolizes GABA. Reducing GABA degradation increases GABA levels. Tiagabine increases GABA levels by blocking the reuptake of GABA by neurons and glia cells, prolonging GABA's effect in the synaptic cleft. Gabapentin was designed as GABA attached to a lipid-soluble ring that facilitates its passage across the blood-brain barrier. Gabapentin appears to increase GABA activity in the brain, but the precise mechanism is unknown. Valproic acid also increases GABA activity. Differences in the mechanisms by which GABA activity is increased by these drugs as well as other non–GABA-related effects explain their different efficacy and side-effect profiles (51).

Since GABA is the principal inhibitory neurotransmitter in the human brain, simply consuming more dietary GABA is a logical way to treat epilepsy. Unfortunately, GABA is a charged molecule with both an amine and carboxylic acid group: it does not readily cross the blood-brain barrier. Increased dietary levels of GABA have minimal effect on brain levels of GABA and do not reduce seizure activity (52). Agents that increase the permeability of the blood-brain barrier, such as nitric oxide or other free radicals, may facilitate dietary GABA supplements in reaching brain tissue but would also increase toxic chemical levels in the brain (52–53). The blood-brain barrier evolved for a reason—to protect the brain from toxins and avoid rapid shifts in the levels of many bioactive substances. Some alternative therapists recommend that GABA be dosed in the range of 500 to 2,000 g/d to treat epilepsy, but it is unclear if any of this therapy reaches the brain or influences seizure activity.

TAURINE

Taurine (2-aminoethanesulfonic acid) is a conditionally essential amino acid because the body needs it and cannot synthesize it on its own. However, taurine is not used for protein synthesis. Often labeled as an amino acid, taurine is technically not an amino acid since it lacks a carboxyl group. Taurine is derived from cysteine; both compounds contain sulfur. Taurine is present in meat, fish, eggs, and dairy products. This molecule is also present in some energy drinks; it is the ingredient from which Red Bull derives its name.

Taurine is involved in several different metabolic processes, including detoxification, cell membrane stabilization, and regulating intracellular calcium levels (54–55). These processes help maintain neuronal activity. Animal studies suggest that taurine can increase inhibitory neurotransmission and help prevent epileptic seizures (56–58). Magnesium-deficient mice with audiogenic seizures were treated with 3 different types of magnesium supplementation: magnesium acetyltaurinate (contained taurine), magnesium pyrrolidine-2-carboxylate, and magnesium chloride (59). Only treatment with magnesium acetyltaurinate showed lasting effects for seizure control. In humans, cerebrospinal fluid taurine levels decline after seizures, while glutamate and aspartate levels rise. Altered plasma and urinary taurine levels have led some to speculate that taurine may have a role in epileptogenesis (60). There are associations between increased taurine levels and reduced seizure susceptibility, and between decreased taurine levels and more spontaneous seizure activity (61). These trends do not establish taurine as an AED (61).

Only a small fraction of plasma taurine crosses the blood-brain barrier. Therefore, dietary taurine supplementation should not significantly alter brain activity. Some practitioners recommend taurine for epilepsy, usually advocating around 2,000 mg/d of taurine. Whether dietary taurine supplementation affects the brain or epilepsy is uncertain. Studies on taurine supplementation (200 mg/d to 21 g/d) for epilepsy found positive and negative effects (62–68). In many of the studies showing positive results, effects are similar to those seen from placebos in double-blind controlled trials. If taurine has short-term benefits in reducing seizures in some patients, the optimal dose is uncertain. Some studies suggest that a range of 100 to 500 mg/d is best for short-term improvements, with loss of efficacy at doses exceeding 1,500 mg/d (69). In several studies, benefits were transient, lasting only a few weeks. These observations do not distinguish a true short-term benefit from a placebo effect. No significant side effects of taurine therapy are known, but there is no evidence that oral taurine reduces or increases seizure activity in humans.

Some alternative practitioners recommend the amino acids L-taurine and L-tyrosine to help control seizures. L-Tyrosine is a critical amino acid in protein synthesis and also forms the building block for several neurotransmitters. There is no evidence that supplementation reduces seizure activity.

CARNITINE

Carnitine is an ammonium compound synthesized from the essential amino acids methionine and lysine. L-Carnitine is the biologically active isomer. It serves as a cofactor in the transportation of long-chain, unbound fatty acids into mitochondria during the breakdown of lipids to generate adenosine triphosphate (energy). We obtain 75% of the carnitine from meat and dairy products, and the rest is synthesized by the body. Carnitine has neuroprotective effects in rodent seizure models (70). However, numerous compounds, including most AEDs, show similar effects, but these have been notoriously difficult to show in humans. Carnitine crosses through the blood-brain barrier via 2 transporters.

Valproic acid inhibits carnitine biosynthesis by decreasing the concentration of α-ketoglutarate, which lowers carnitine concentrations (71–72). Carnitine supplementation may increase the beta-oxidation of valproic acid, thereby limiting cytosolic omega-oxidation and production of toxic metabolites of valproic acid that may cause liver toxicity and hyperammonemia. Since L-carnitine is safe, it is often recommended in cases with valproic acid toxicity or poisoning, especially in children. However, the protection of hepatic tissue or shortening duration of depressed level of consciousness remains suggestive based on available but inconclusive studies (73). Prophylactic carnitine supplementation is often recommended during valproic acid (VPA) therapy in high-risk pediatric patients, such as those younger than 2 years or those with known metabolic disorders or carnitine deficiency states (74–75). In 1998, a panel of pediatric neurologists recommended carnitine supplementation for patients with specific carnitine deficiency syndromes, especially infants and children on long-term VPA treatment (74).

Carnitine deficiency can cause fatigue, muscle weakness, enlarged heart, irregular heartbeat, frequent infection, seizures, poor muscle tone, slow growth, chronic vomiting, chronic fever, hyperammonemia, and hypoglycemia. Isolated reports suggest that carnitine supplementation can reduce valproate side effects, such as tremor and tiredness, but controlled studies show no benefit (76). A double-blind, placebo-controlled crossover study on 47 children taking valproic acid or carbamazepine found no difference in parental reports of improved seizure control or reduced side effects with carnitine supplementation (76). Given the cost and lack of proven effect, routine supplementation with L-carnitine is not recommended in older children and adults taking VPA.

CARNOSINE

Carnosine is a dipeptide of the amino acids histidine and β-alanine. Carnosine is most abundant in muscle and brain tissues. Carnosine has antioxidant properties and modulates neuronal levels of zinc and copper (77). It is most easily found and measured as homocarnosine, a dipeptide metabolite of GABA and histidine. Carnosine shows antiepileptic efficacy in animal models (78–79).

It is unclear if carnosine or homocarnosine is directly involved with seizure activity in humans or if their supplementation alters seizure control (80). Children with uncontrolled epilepsy and febrile seizures have higher homocarnosine levels than those with controlled epilepsy (81). Homocarnosine levels are higher in patients who respond to AED therapy (82–84). Parallel increases in homocarnosine and GABA levels may follow AED therapy. Homocarnosine levels vary with GABA levels but do not necessarily correlate directly with seizure control (80, 84). A magnetic resonance spectroscopy study found that patients with juvenile myoclonic epilepsy had normal levels of homocarnosine and those with complex partial seizures had lower levels of homocarnosine. Higher homocarnosine levels correlated with better seizure control in both groups (85). An unblinded study showed reduced epileptiform activity in the EEGs of 5 of 7 patients who received dietary supplements of carnosine for 10 weeks (77). Blinded therapists reported improved cognition, behavior, and language function on informal assessments. This group also showed improvements with carnosine supplementation in autism (86). Neither study has been replicated. More rigorous studies are needed to confirm or refute these findings in small pilot studies. The role of homocarnosine as a therapeutic agent for epilepsy remains unproven but warrants further study.

GLYCINE AND DIMETHYLGLYCINE

Glycine is the simplest of amino acids and acts as an inhibitory neurotransmitter in the central nervous system. Different forms of glycine have been tested for their anticonvulsant properties. One animal study found that trimethylglycine, dimethylglycine (DMG), and methylglycine reduced the number of seizures induced by strychnine (87). A randomized clinical trial of 19 institutionalized patients found DMG had no effect on seizure frequency compared with placebo (88). Most literature reports that dimethylglycine has no significant therapeutic effect in reducing seizure activity in humans (89–90). However, some researchers suggest that, in selected individuals, DMG supplementation at 100 mg twice a day may have some benefit (91).

Dimethylglycine is a derivative of the amino acid glycine. Once postulated as a vitamin (B_{16}), it is now considered a food product since no ill effects of DMG deficiency are known. Dimethylglycine is found in liver and beans and can be purchased as a supplement. Animal studies have shown conflicting results about DMG, with one showing that DMG has anticonvulsant properties and another showing that it does not (87, 89).

MINERALS

Minerals are inorganic elements that are essential nutrients for various bodily functions. There are 16 essential minerals that are critical for the body to function. For example, bone growth and maintenance requires calcium, and blood oxygenation depends on iron. Trace elements such as zinc, copper, and manganese have important roles in the nervous system. Genetic selenium deficiency states in animals can lead to seizures (92). Other genetically seizure-prone animals show alterations in brain zinc, selenium, and cobalt concentrations. This suggests that the homeostastis of these minerals is involved in susceptibility, development, or termination of seizures (93). One study found that average copper, magnesium, and zinc levels in hair were significantly lower in people with epilepsy than controls (94). The authors suggest that, in such patients, these minerals should be supplemented. Serum analysis showed no differences in the average magnesium and zinc levels between patients treated with AEDs and those not receiving drug therapy. These animal studies and preliminary clinical findings suggest that AED therapy does not impact trace mineral levels; it is the condition of epilepsy, underlying causes, or other factors that cause these differences. However, further replication is needed.

Very low levels of sodium, calcium, and magnesium can alter the electrical activity of brain cells and cause seizures. Dietary deficiency of these minerals is rare unless there is severe malnutrition. However, other factors can affect the levels in the body. Low sodium levels can result from medications (e.g., diuretics, carbamazepine, or oxcarbazepine), excessive water intake, or hormonal disorders. Low calcium levels can result from kidney disease or hormonal disorders. Individuals who chronically abuse alcohol and have poor nutrition from diet or illness (e.g., cancer, HIV/AIDS) can develop low magnesium levels, and this can secondarily lower calcium levels, as well.

People with epilepsy seldom need mineral supplementation for seizure control. Changes in diet or mineral supplements are advised if levels of these minerals are low. Antiepileptic drugs that increase or alter liver metabolism (e.g., carbamazepine, phenobarbital, phenytoin, primidone, and valproate) can increase vitamin D metabolism, thereby lowering serum vitamin D levels. This may cause osteopenia or osteoporosis. Combined calcium and vitamin D supplementation may help prevent bone loss. Vitamin D levels should be obtained in patients taking these drugs. A bone density test can detect this possible complication. If significant reduction of bone density (osteopenia) is found, consultation with a bone metabolism specialist can help.

Magnesium is needed for calcium absorption, and the ratio of calcium to magnesium affects neuronal functions. Magnesium is abundant in green vegetables, nuts, seeds, and some whole grains. Mild magnesium deficiency occurs in some people with epilepsy and may contribute to increased seizure susceptibility (95). Pilot, unblinded studies suggest that magnesium supplements (450 mg/d) can improve seizure control (96). It remains uncertain if magnesium supplements can reduce seizures in specific populations with epilepsy, such as those with slightly low serum magnesium levels. Notably, magnesium sulfate is the treatment of choice for preventing the progression of severe preeclampsia and in preventing recurrent convulsions in eclampsia (97).

Zinc deficiency is rare and usually results from severe nutritional compromise or an inherited defect in zinc absorption. However, AED use can occasionally cause zinc deficiency in a small number of patients (98–100). Zinc deficiency increases seizure susceptibility in animal models of epilepsy (101). Zinc and copper have an antagonistic relationship. Zinc levels are lower in people with epilepsy, and the use of AEDs may also contribute to zinc deficiency. Zinc supplements of 15 to 50mg/d is an appropriate adult dose.

Copper is important in the physiology of red blood cells as well as the immune, neurologic, and skeletal systems. Good sources of dietary copper are shellfish (especially oysters), organ meats (liver, kidney), whole grains, nuts, raisins, legumes, and chocolate.

Copper deficiency may cause seizures; however, in patients treated for epilepsy, copper levels are elevated, possibly owing to copper complexes formed by the activation of AEDs or a primary effect of the process that causes seizures (102). The ratio of zinc to copper may influence health and seizure susceptibility. Copper appears to have oxidant and zinc antioxidant properties (103). One theory holds that seizures are more likely to occur when the copper-zinc ratio increases suddenly in the relative absence of taurine (91). There are little experimental data and less clinical data to support this. A 1:10 to 1:30 to ratio of copper to zinc is recommended (104). Elevated ratios are common with aging and illness (103). Copper supplements of 1 to 3 mg/d are appropriate for adults.

Some side effects of valproate may be prevented by mineral supplementation. Inflammation of the pancreas (pancreatitis), which is a rare but serious adverse effect of valproate, may be prevented by selenium supplementation. Selenium at a dose of 100 μg/d was used to prevent valproate-induced pancreatitis in a child who previously had this problem when taking valproate. Selenium (10–20 μg/d), zinc (30–50 mg/d), and biotin (1,000–2,500 μcg/d) may help counteract hair loss that can result from valproate use. These doses are available in many over-the-counter, high-potency multivitamins.

Manganese toxicity or deficiency can rarely cause seizures. Manganese toxicity can result from excess manganese supplementation, in which case it quickly resolves when supplements are discontinued (105). Manganese deficiency is more common than toxicity and results from a paucity of manganese-rich foods, such as grain products, nuts, legumes, and leafy greens. Average daily intake in the United States from food sources is 3 mg. Manganese supplementation is typically recommended at 2 to 5 mg/d. An old Anglo-Saxon prescription for "devil sickness" (epilepsy) was lupine, a plant exceptionally high in manganese (106). Serum manganese levels are low in people with epilepsy and do not appear to result from AEDs (107–108). No studies have systematically assessed manganese supplementation on seizure control.

OMEGA FATTY ACIDS

Fats have received an undeservedly bad reputation in the United States. They are falsely convicted of causing the epidemic of obesity, diabetes, and hypercholesterolemia. Carbohydrates are now recognized as the prime culprits of the rampant rise of obesity and diabetes and are significant contributors to elevated cholesterol levels. Fats provide calories as well as essential compounds for the normal functioning of our bodies. Fats can be unhealthy, but it is the type of fat and the quantity that matter.

Simplistically, monounsaturated and polyunsaturated fatty acids are healthy, while saturated and trans fats are unhealthy. The saturated hydrogenated fats are associated with increased rates of cardiovascular disease, diabetes, cancer, and degenerative diseases (e.g., Alzheimer disease) (109–111). Fat makes up nearly 60% of the brain, and fat critically contributes to brain structure and function—but which fats are key? Instead of focusing on the amount of fat consumed, the mix of fats may be more important.

Polyunsaturated fatty acids are an essential component of neuronal cell membranes and also function in the normal physiology of many other organ systems. These are essential fatty acids; we must consume them since our bodies are unable to synthesize these compounds. The essential fatty acids are involved in growth, cell division, energy production, neuronal and immunologic function, oxygen transfer from the air to blood, and hemoglobin synthesis. Two important essential fatty acids are ω-3 and ω-6. ω-3 fatty acids have antiinflammatory properties, while ω-6 fatty acids have proinflammatory properties. Diets consumed by hunter-gatherers, from whom we recently (12,000 years ago) evolved, contained a more balanced ratio of these fatty acids. Similarly, the Mediterranean diet, associated with lower rates of cardiovascular disease and longevity, has a more balanced ratio of these fatty acids. By contrast, Western diets of corn-fed meat and large amounts high-glycemic carbohydrates (e.g., sugars, processed grains) shift the ratio toward ω-6 fatty acids.

ω-3 fatty acids have neuroprotective properties in animal models of stroke and also raise the seizure threshold (112–113). Other animal models have demonstrated the potential for fatty acids rich in ω-3 to improve reduce seizure activity (114). However, as noted above, a trial of ω-3 fatty acids in patients with treatment-resistant epilepsy showed no benefits. It is possible that longer trials, different doses, other supplements, or lifestyle changes may be needed to detect a beneficial effect of ω-3 fatty acids in human epilepsy.

CONCLUSION

Nutritional therapies remain an attractive naturalistic approach to controlling epilepsy. Apart from the ketogenic and modified Atkins diets and very rare disorders such as pyridoxine-deficient seizures, no dietary changes or supplements are known to improve seizure control in people with epilepsy. Similarly, there is no clear evidence that any foods or supplements increase seizure activity. Nutrition, the most fundamental aspect of health, remains a largely uncharted domain in the health of individuals with epilepsy.

It is tempting, given the effectiveness of the ketogenic and modified Atkins diets in helping to control seizures, to speculate that a lower-carbohydrate diet may reduce seizures and a high-carbohydrate diet may increase seizures. But there is no solid evidence to support or refute these claims. They are worth exploring in the future with well-controlled studies.

We recommend a balanced diet that includes all of the essential nutrients. Since any physical or emotional stress can make seizures more likely to occur, we advocate a diet that meets the energetic, fluid, and special needs of any individual with epilepsy. Since some medications, such as carbamazepine, can elevate serum lipid levels and predispose to cardiovascular disease, other aspects of nutrition should also be addressed in people with epilepsy. What about supplements? There are many vitamins, amino acids, and minerals recommended for people with epilepsy, but we need more information to understand their role.

REFERENCES

1. Barlow S, Schlatter J. Risk assessment of carcinogens in food. *Toxicol Appl Pharmacol.* 2010;243:180–190.
2. Bouchard MF, Bellinger DC, Wright RO, et al. Attention-deficit/hyperactivity disorder and urinary metabolites of organophosphate pesticides. *Pediatrics.* 2010;125:1270–1277.
3. Taubes G. *Good Calories, Bad Calories.* New York, NY: Random House; 2007:89–90.
4. American Dietetic Association. Position of the American Dietetic Association: functional foods. *J Am Dietetic Assoc.* 2009;109:735–746.
5. Westman EC, Yancy WS, Edman JS, et al. Effect of 6-month adherence to a very low carbohydrate diet program. *Am J Med.* 2002;113(1):30–36.
6. Freeman JM, Vining EP. Seizures decrease rapidly after fasting: preliminary studies of the ketogenic diet. *Arch Pediatr Adolesc Med.* 1999;153(9):946–949.
7. Mahoney AW, Hendricks DG, Bernhard N, et al. Fasting and ketogenic diet effects on audiogenic seizures susceptibility of magnesium deficient rats. *Pharmacol Biochem Behav.* 1983;18(5):683–687.
8. Malouf R, Brust JC. Hypoglycemia: causes, neurological manifestations, and outcome. *Ann Neurol.* 1985;17(5):421–430.
9. Naritoku DK. Hypoglycemia and seizures. http://www.siumed.edu/neuro/epilepsy/QNA/QNAframes/hypoglycemiajs.html. Accessed April 4, 2003.
10. Gropman AL. Diagnosis and treatment of childhood mitochondria diseases. *Curr Neurol Neurosci Rep.* 2001;1(2):185–194.
11. Gold DR, Cohn BH. Treatment of mitochondria cytopathies. *Semin Neurol.* 2001;21(3):309–325.
12. Butchko HH, Stargel WW, Comer CP, et al. Aspartame: review of safety. *Regul Toxicol Pharmacol.* 2002;35(2Pt2):S1–93
13. Rowan AJ, Shaywitz BA, Tuchman L, et al. Aspartame and seizure susceptibility: results of a clinical study in reportedly sensitive individuals. *Epilepsia.* 1995;36(3):270–275.
14. Ogunmekan AO, Hwan PA. A randomized, double-blind, placebo-controlled, clinical trial of D-alpha-tocopheryl acetate (vitamin E), as add-on therapy, for epilepsy in children. *Epilepsia.* 1989;30:84–89.
15. Ogunmekan AO. Vitamin E deficiency and seizures in animals and man. *Can J Neurol Sci.* 1979;6:43–45.
16. Schlanger S, Shinitzky M, Yam D. Diet enriched with omega-3 fatty acids alleviates convulsion symptoms in epilepsy patients. *Epilepsia.* 2002;43(1):103–104.
17. Maynard M, Gunnell D, Emmett P, et al. Fruit, vegetables, and antioxidants in childhood and risk of adult cancer: the Boyd Orr cohort. *J Epidemiol Community Health.* 2003;57(3):218–225.
18. Weisburger JH. Lifestyle, health and disease prevention: the underlying mechanisms. *Eur J Cancer Prev.* 2002;11(suppl 2):S1–7.
19. Freeman JM, Vining EP, Pillas DJ. The efficacy of the ketogenic diet—1998: a prospective evaluation of intervention in 150 children. *Pediatrics.* 1998;102:1358–1363.
20. Neal EG, Chaffe H, Schwartz RH. The ketogenic diet for the treatment of childhood epilepsy: a randomised control trial. *Lancet Neurol.* 2008;7:500–506.
21. Neal EG, Chaffe H, Schwartz RH et al. A randomized trial of classical and medium-chain triglyceride ketogenic diets in the treatment of childhood epilepsy. *Epilepsia.* 2009;50:1109–1117.
22. Nylen K, Likhodii S, Burnham WM. The ketogenic diet: proposed mechanisms of action. *Neurotherapeutics.* 2009;6:402–405.

23. Kossoff EH, Zupec-Kania BA, Rho JM. Ketogenic diets: an update for child neurologists. *J Child Neurol.* 2009;24:979–988.

24. Kossoff EH, Zupec-Kania BA, Amark PE, et al. Optimal clinical management of children receiving the ketogenic diet: recommendations of the International Ketogenic Diet Study Group. *Epilepsia.* 2009;50:304–317.

25. Kossoff EH, Zupec-Kania BA, Amark PE, et al. Optimal clinical management of children receiving the ketogenic diet: recommendations of the International Ketogenic Diet Study Group. *Epilepsia.* 2009;50:304–317.

26. Hong AM, Turner Z, Hamdy RF, et al. Infantile spasms treated with the ketogenic diet: prospective single-center experience in 104 consecutive infants. *Epilepsia.* 2010;51(8): 1403–1407.

27. Kossoff EH, Laux LC, Blackford R, et al. When do seizures improve with the ketogenic diet? *Epilepsia.* 2008;49:329–333.

28. Bergqvist AG, Schall JI, Gallagher PR, et al. Fasting versus gradual initiation of the ketogenic diet: a prospective, randomized clinical trial of efficacy. *Epilepsia.* 2005;46: 1810–1819.

29. Seo JH, Lee YM, Lee JS, et al. Efficacy and tolerability of the ketogenic diet according to the lipid:nonlipid ratios—comparison of 3:1 with 4:1 diet. *Epilepsia.* 2007;48:801–805.

30. Henderson CB, Filloux FM, Alder SC, et al. Efficacy of the ketogenic diet as a treatment option for epilepsy: meta-analysis. *J Child Neurol.* 2006;21:193–198.

31. McNally MA, Pyzik PL, Rubenstein JE, et al. Empiric use of potassium citrate reduces kidney-stone incidence with the ketogenic diet. *Pediatrics.* 2009;124:e300–304.

32. Mostovsky DI, Yehuda S. The use of fatty acids in the diet for seizure management. In: Devinsky O, Schachter S, Pacia S, eds. *Complementary and Alternate Therapies for Epilepsy.* New York, NY: Demos Medical Publishing; 2005:205–218.

33. Bromfield E, Dworetzky B, Hurwitz S, et al. A randomized trial of polyunsaturated fatty acids for refractory epilepsy. *Epilepsy Behav.* 2008;12:187–190.

34. Hurrell R. Influence of vegetable protein sources on trace element and mineral bioavailability. *J Nutr.* 2003;133:2973S–2977S.

35. Omenn G, Goodman G, Thornquist M, et al. Risk factors for lung cancer and for intervention effects in CARET, the Beta-Carotene and Retinol Efficacy Trial. *J Natl Cancer Insti.* 1996;88:1550–1559.

36. Albanes D. Beta-carotene and lung cancer: a case study. *Am J Clin Nutr.* 1999;69: 1345S–1350S.

37. Bjelakovic G, Nikolova D, Gluud L, Simonetti R, Gluud C. Mortality in randomized trials of antioxidant supplements for primary and secondary prevention: systematic review and meta-analysis. *JAMA.* 2007;297:842–857.

38. Sudha K, Rao AV, Rao A. Oxidative stress and antioxidants in epilepsy. *Clinica Chimica Acta.* 2001;303:19–24.

39. Waldbaum S, Patel M. Mitochondria, oxidative stress, and temporal lobe epilepsy. *Epilepsy Res.* 2010;88:23–45.

40. Kim do Y, Rho JM. The ketogenic diet and epilepsy. *Curr Opin Clin Nutr Metab Care.* 2008;11:113–120.

41. Raju GB, Behari M, Prasad K, Ahuja GK. Randomized, double-blind, placebo-controlled, clinical trial of D-alpha-tocopherol (vitamin E) as add-on therapy in uncontrolled epilepsy. *Epilepsia.* 1994;35:368–372.

42. Ogunmekan AO. Plasma vitamin E (alpha tocopherol) levels in normal children and in epileptic children with and without anticonvulsant drug therapy. *Trop Geogr Med.* 1985;37:175–7. Hung-Ming W, Liu CS, Tsai JJ, Ko LY, Wei YH. Antioxidant and anticonvulsant effect of a modified formula of chaihu-longu-muli-tang. *Am J Chin Med.* 2002;30:339–346.

43. Hung-Ming W, Liu CS, Tsai JJ, Ko LY, Wei YH. Antioxidant and anticonvulsant effect of a modified formula of chaihu-longu-muli-tang. *AM J Chin Med.* 2002;30:339–346.
44. Major P, Greenberg E, Khan A, Thiele EA. Pyridoxine supplementation for the treatment of levetiracetam-induced behavior side effects in children: preliminary results. *Epilepsy Behav.* 2008;13:557–559.
45. Dordain G, Deffond D. Pyridoxine neuropathies: review of the literature. *Therapie.* 1994;49:333–337.
46. Morra M, Philipszoon HD, D'Andrea G, Cananzi AR, L'Erario R, Milone FF. Sensory and motor neuropathy caused by excessive ingestion of vitamin B_6: a case report. *Funct Neurol.* 1993;8:429–432.
47. Gupta VK, Mishra D, Mathur I, Singh KK. Pyridoxine-dependent seizures: a case report and a critical review of the literature. *J Paediatr Child Health.* 2001;37:592–596.
48. Plecko B, Stöckler S. Vitamin B_6 dependent seizures. *Can J Neurol Sci.* 2009;36(suppl 2): S73–S77.
49. Raevskii KS, Avakian GN, Kudrin VS, Nesterova SI, Gusev EI. Features of neurotransmitter pool in cerebrospinal fluid of patients with epilepsy. *Zh Nevrol Psikhiatr Im S S Korsakova.* 2001;101:39–41.
50. Czuczwar SJ, Patsalos PN. The new generation of GABA enhancers: potential in the treatment of epilepsy. *CNS Drugs.* 2001;15:339–350.
51. Treiman DM. GABAergic mechanisms in epilepsy. *Epilepsia.* 2001;42(suppl 3):8–12.
52. Shyamaladevi N, Jayakumar AR, Sujatha R, Paul V, Subramanian EH. Evidence that nitric oxide production increases γ-amino butyric acid permeability of blood-brain barrier. *Brain Res Bull.* 2002;57:231–236.
53. Oztas B, Kilic S, Dural E, Ispir T. Influence of antioxidants on the blood-brain barrier permeability during epileptic seizures. *J Neurosci Res.* 2001;66:674–678.
54. Birdsall TC. Therapeutic applications of taurine. *Altern Med Rev.* 1998;3:128–136.
55. Baran H. Alterations of taurine in the brain of chronic kainic acid epilepsy model. *Amino Acids.* 2006;31:303–307.
56. Rainesalo S, Keränen T, Palmio J, Peltola J, Oja SS, Saransaari P. Plasma and cerebrospinal fluid amino acids in epileptic patients. *Neurochem Res.* 2004; 29:319–324.
57. El Idrissi A, Messing J, Scalia J, Trenkner E. Prevention of epileptic seizures by taurine. *Adv Exp Med Biol.* 2003;526:515–525.
58. Junyent F, Utrera J, Romero R, et al. Prevention of epilepsy by taurine treatments in mice experimental model. *J Neurosci Res.* 2009;87:1500–1508.
59. Bac P, Herrenknecht C, Binet P, Durlach J. Audiogenic seizures in magnesium-deficient mice: effects of magnesium pyrrolidone-2-carboxylate, magnesium acetyltaurinate, magnesium chloride and vitamin B-6. *Magnes Res.* 1983;6:11–19.
60. Collins BW, Goodman HO, Swanton CH, Remy CN. Plasma and urinary taurine in epilepsy. *Clin Chem.* 1988;34:671–675.
61. Durelli L, Mutani R. The current status of taurine in epilepsy. *Clin Neuropharmacol.* 1983;6:37–48.
62. Bergamini L, Mutani R, Delsedime M, Durelli L. First clinical experience on the antiepileptic action of taurine. *Eur Neurol.* 1974;11:261–269.
63. Pennetta R, Masi G, Perniola T, Ferrannini E. Electroclinical evaluation of the antiepileptic action of taurine. *Acta Neurol (Napoli).* 1977;32:316–322.
64. Takahashi R, Nakane Y. Clinical trial of taurine in epilepsy. In: Barbeau A, Huxtable RJ, eds. *Taurine and Neurological Disorders.* New York, NY: Raven Press; 1978:375–385.
65. Konig P, Kriechbaum G, Presslich O, Schubert H, Schuster P, Sieghart W. Orally-administered taurine in therapy-resistant epilepsy. *Wien Klin Wochenschr.* 1977;89: 111–113.
66. Barbeau A, Donaldson J. Zinc, taurine, and epilepsy. *Arch Neurol.* 1974;30:52–58.

67. Fukuyama Y, Ochiai Y. Therapeutic trial by taurine for intractable childhood epilepsies. *Brain Dev.* 1982;4:63–69.

68. Mantovani J, DeVivo DC. Effects of taurine on seizures and growth hormone release in epileptic patients. *Arch Neurol.* 1979;36:672–674.

69. Gaby AR. Natural approaches to epilepsy. *Alt Med Rev.* 2007;12:9–24.

70. Igisu H, Matsuoka M, Iryo Y. Protection of the brain by carnitine. *Sangyo Eiseigaku Zasshi.* 1995;37:75–82.

71. Thom H, Carter PE, Cole GF, Stevenson KL. Ammonia and carnitine concentrations in children treated with sodium valproate compared with other anticonvulsant drugs. *Dev Med Child Neurol.* 1991;33:795–802.

72. Van Wouwe JP. Carnitine deficiency during valproic acid treatment. *Int J Vitam Nutr Res.* 1995;65:211–214.

73. Lheureux PE, Hantson P. Carnitine in the treatment of valproic acid–induced toxicity. *Clin Toxicol.* 2009;47:101–111.

74. DeVivo DC, Bohan TP, Coulter DL, et al. L-Carnitine supplementation in childhood epilepsy: current perspectives. *Epilepsia.* 1998;39:1216–1225.

75. Coulter DL. Carnitine, valproate, and toxicity. *J Child Neurol.* 1991;6:7–14.

76. Freeman JM, Vining EP, Cost S, Singhi P. Does carnitine administration improve the symptoms attributed to anticonvulsant medications?: A double-blinded crossover study. *Pediatrics.* 1994;93(6Pt1):893–895.

77. Chez MG, Buchanan CP, Komen JL. L-carnosine therapy for intractable epilepsy in childhood: effect on EEG. *Epilepsia.* 2002;43:65.

78. Wu XH, Ding MP, Zhu-Ge ZB, Zhu YY, Jin CL, Chen Z. Carnosine, a precursor of histidine, ameliorates pentylenetetrazole-induced kindled seizures in rat. *Neurosci Lett.* 2006;400:146–149.

79. Kozan R, Sefil F, Bağirici F. Anticonvulsant effect of carnosine on penicillin-induced epileptiform activity in rats. *Brain Res.* 2008;1239:249–255.

80. Henry TR, Theodore WH. Homocarnosine elevations: a cause or a sign of seizure control? *Neurology.* 2001;56:698–699.

81. Takahashi H. Studies on homocarnosine in cerebrospinal fluid in infancy and childhood. Part II. Homocarnosine levels in cerebrospinal fluid from children with epilepsy, febrile convulsions or meningitis. *Brain Dev.* 1981;3:263–270.

82. Petroff OA, Hyder F, Collins T, Mattson RH, Rothman DL. Acute effects of vigabatrin on brain GABA and homocarnosine in patients with complex partial seizures. *Epilepsia.* 1999;40:958–964.

83. Petroff OA, Hyder F, Rothman DL, Mattson RH. Effects of gabapentin on brain GABA, homocarnosine, and pyrrolidinone in epilepsy patients. *Epilepsia.* 2000;41:675–680.

84. Pitkanen A, Matilainen R, Ruutiainen T, Riekkinen P. Levels of total gamma-aminobutyric acid (GABA), free GABA and homocarnosine in cerebrospinal fluid of epileptic patients before and during gamma-vinyl-GABA (vigabatrin) treatment. *J Neurol Sci.* 1988;88: 83–93.

85. Petroff OA, Hyder F, Rothman DL, Mattson RH. Homocarnosine and seizure control in juvenile myoclonic epilepsy and complex partial seizures. *Neurology.* 2001;56:709–715.

86. Chez MG, Buchanan CP, Aimonovitch MC, et al. Double-blind, placebo-controlled study of L-carnosine supplementation in children with autistic spectrum disorders. *J Child Neurol.* 2002;17:833–837.

87. Freed WJ. Prevention of strychnine-induced seizures and death by the N-methylated glycine derivatives betaine, dimethylglycine and sarcosine. *Pharmacol Biochem Behav.* 1985;22:641–643.

88. Gascon G, Patterson B, Yearwood K, Slotnick H. N,N dimethylglycine and epilepsy. *Epilepsia.* 1989;30:90–93.

89. Haidukewych D, Rodin EA. N,N-dimethylglycine shows no anticonvulsant potential. *Ann Neurol.* 1984;15:405.

90. Roach ES, Gibson P. Failure of N,N-dimethylglycine in epilepsy. *Ann Neurol.* 1983; 14:347.

91. Department of Neurology, Massachusetts General Hospital. Epilepsy and nutritional supplementation. http://neuro-www.mgh.harvard.edu/forum/EpilepsyF/11.22.973.29AM EpilepsyNutrition. Accessed April 4, 2003.

92. Schweizer U, Bräuer AU, Köhrle J, Nitsch R, Savaskan NE. Selenium and brain function: a poorly recognized liaison. *Brain Res Brain Res Rev.* 2004;45:164–78.

93. Hirate M, Takeda A, Tamano H, Enomoto S, Oku N. Distribution of trace elements in the brain of EL (epilepsy) mice. *Epilepsy Res.* 2002;51:109–116.

94. Ilhan A, Uz E, Kali S, Var A, Akyol O. Serum and hair trace element levels in patients with epilepsy and healthy subjects: does the antiepileptic therapy affect the element of concentrations of hair? *Eur J Neurol.* 1999;6:705–709.

95. Leaver DD, Parkinson GB, Schneider KM. Neurologic consequences of magnesium deficiency: correlations with epilepsy. *Clin Exp Pharm Physiol.* 2007;14:361–370.

96. Murphy P. Magnesium and manganese: raising the seizure threshold. *Epilepsy Wellness Newsletter.* Spring 1999.

97. Sibai BM. Diagnosis, prevention, and management of eclampsia. *Obstet Gynecol.* 2005; 105:402–410.

98. Lewis-Jones MS, Evans S, Culshaw MA. Cutaneous manifestations of zinc deficiency during treatment with anticonvulsants. *Br Med J.* 1985;290:603–604.

99. Schott GD, Delves HT. Plasma zinc levels with anticonvulsant therapy. *Br J Clin Pharmacol.* 1978;5:279–280.

100. Verrotti A, Basciani F, Trotta D, Pomilio MP, Morgese G, Chiarelli F. Serum copper, zinc, selenium, glutathione peroxidase levels in epileptic children before and after 1 year of sodium valproate and carbamazepine therapy. *Epilepsy Res.* 2002;48:71–75.

101. Fukahori M, Itoh M. Effects of dietary zinc status on seizure susceptibility and hippocampal zinc content in the EI (epilepsy) mouse. *Brain Res.* 1990;529:16–22.

102. Brunia CHM, Buyze G. Serum copper levels in epilepsy. *Epilepsia.* 1972;13:621–625.

103. Mezzetti A, Pierdomenico SD, Costantini F, et al. Copper/zinc ratio and systemic oxidant load: effect of aging and aging-related degenerative diseases. *Free Radic Biol Med.* 1998;25:676–681.

104. Haas EM. Zinc. http://www.healthy.net/asp/templates/article.asp?PageType=article&ID= 2071. Accessed April 4, 2003.

105. Komaki H, Maisawa S, Sugai K, Kobayashi Y, Hashimoto T. Tremor and seizures associated with chronic manganese intoxication. *Brain Dev.* 1999;21:122–124.

106. Dendle P. Lupines, manganese, and devil-sickness: an Anglo-Saxon medical response to epilepsy. *Bull Hist Med.* 2001;75:91–101.

107. Papavasiliou PS, Kutt H, Miller ST, Rosal V, Wang YY, Aronson RB. Manganese tissue levels in treated epileptics. *Neurology.* 1979;29:1466–1473.

108. Carl GF, Keen CL, Gallagher BB, et al. Association of low blood manganese concentrations in epilepsy. *Neurology.* 1986;36:1584–1587.

109. Cernea S, Hâncu N, Raz I. Diet and coronary heart disease in diabetes. *Acta Diabetol.* 2003;40(suppl 2):S389–400.

110. Gillette Guyonnet S, Abellan Van Kan G, Andrieu S, et al. IANA task force on nutrition and cognitive decline with aging. *J Nutr Health Aging.* 2007;11:132–152.

111. Trichopoulou A, Lagiou P. Worldwide patterns of dietary lipids intake and health implications. *Am J Clin Nutr.* 1997;66(4 suppl):961S–964S.

112. Blondeau N, Widmann C, Lazdunski M, Heurteaux C. Polyunsaturated fatty acids induce ischemic and epileptic intolerance. *Neurosci.* 2002;109:231–241.

113. Rabinovitz S, Mostofsky DI, Yehuda S. Anticonvulsant efficiency, behavioral performance, and cortisol levels: a comparison of carbamazapine and a fatty acid compound. *Psychoendocrinology.* 2004;29:113–124.

114. Yehuda S, Rabinovitz S, Carasso RL, Mostofsky DI. The role of polyunsaturated fatty acids in restoring the aging neuronal membrane. *Neurobiol Aging.* 2002;23:843–53.

4

Alternative Pharmacologic Therapies for Epilepsy

Antiepileptic drugs (AEDs) reduce spontaneous electrical firing in hyperexcitable neurons, thereby preventing initiation and spread of seizures. Traditional AEDs approved by the U.S. Food and Drug Administration (FDA) must demonstrate efficacy in accepted animal models prior to clinical trials and approval for human use. The prevention or control of seizures in animals, produced by electrical stimulation of the brain or by the administration of the proconvulsants, such as pentylenetetrazol, provides direct evidence of a drug's anticonvulsant potential. Following animal studies, AEDs undergo extensive and costly double-blind, controlled clinical investigations prior to approval for human use. For the vast majority of patients, FDA-approved AEDs should always be the first line of defense to prevent and control seizures.

Although there are more than a dozen FDA-approved AEDs, up to 40% of patients still have seizures even with proper dosing and compliance with AED therapy (1). Occasionally, medically refractory patients report improved seizure control after treatment with a medication used for an unrelated indication, such as insomnia, depression, or inflammation. No sufficiently powered double-blind, randomized studies or controlled studies have established the safety or efficacy for the "off-label" uses of these medications in epilepsy. However, for patients with ongoing, disabling seizures that are not controlled by AEDs, it may be reasonable to consider the use of these drugs with careful medical supervision. Table 4.1 lists the many classes of medicines claimed to offer protection from seizures.

ANTIDEPRESSANTS

Depression and anxiety are common in people with epilepsy. However, some physicians prescribe antidepressant medications cautiously in people with epilepsy

61

Table 4.1 Alternative Medications for Epilepsy

Medication Class	FDA-Approved Uses	Examples	Potential Antiepileptic Mechanism
Antidepressants	Depression/ anxiety		
SSRI		Citalopram, fluoxetine	Elevates 5-HT
SNRI		Venlafaxine, duloxetine	Elevates 5-HT > NE
NSRI		Milnacipran	Elevates NE and 5-HT
Immunomodualtory/ anti-inflammatory	Numerous auto-immune and allergic disorders	Prednisone, dexamethasone, intravenous γ-globulin	Stabilizes neuronal membranes, reduces brain's inflammatory and immune response, reduces neuronal antibody response
Carbonic anhydrase inhibitor	Congestive heart failure, glaucoma, altitude sickness, petit mal/unlocalized	Acetazolamide	Reduces pH

for fear of inducing seizures or compounding AED side effects. As a result, and because of widespread underrecognition, people with epilepsy and depression often have untreated mood disorders (2). Consequently, understanding the risks and benefits of antidepressants and their relationship to seizure control is crucial.

Prior to the introduction of selective serotonin reuptake inhibitors (SSRIs), the mainstay of pharmacologic treatment of depression was tricyclic antidepressants (TCAs) and monoamine oxidase inhibitors. Tricyclic antidepressants have mild proconvulsant effects in animals, though controlled studies have never been performed to substantiate this clinical observation. Imipramine, maprotiline, and clomipramine, when used at high doses or titrated, seem to rapidly provoke seizures, while doxepin and the monoamine oxidase inhibitors are considered less proconvulsant (3).

After SSRIs replaced TCAs as first-line medical therapy for depression, seizures following initiation of therapy with SSRIs occurred at a lower rate than with TCAs (4). Moreover, some animal studies support an anticonvulsant effect for the SSRI fluoxetine (Prozac) (5–6). In humans, while overdoses of fluoxetine may result in seizures, some evidence has emerged for an antiepileptic effect at therapeutic doses, either alone or as potentiation of the anticonvulsant effects of traditional AEDs (7). A small unblinded clinical study was performed on 17 patients: fluoxetine 20mg/d was added to the AED of Carbamazepine and phenobarbital, or valproic acid and phenobarbital. Seizures in six of the medically refractory patients came under complete control, and the remainder were reported to have an improvement in seizure frequency. Unfortunately, these encouraging findings have not been reproduced in any larger-scale or double-blind studies. Additionally, any positive effect of fluoxetine on seizure control may have resulted indirectly from fluoxetine's inhibition of hepatic metabolism, thereby increasing the serum concentrations of the AEDs. Further, some people with epilepsy with comorbid depression may experience a reduction of depressive or anxiety symptoms and improved sleep on SSRIs, thus improving seizure control by one of these mechanisms. Numerous other SSRIs have been released since fluoxetine, but none has been well studied for potential anticonvulsant effects. Notably, among 57 people with epilepsy, use of psychotropic medications (14% TCAs, 55% SSRIs, 9% another antidepressant, 9% buspirone, and 3% stimulant) was associated with the following changes in seizure frequency: decreased in 33% of patients, unchanged in 44%, and increased in 23% (8).

A meta-analysis of FDA Phase II and III clinical trials investigated seizure incidence in trials of psychotropic drugs approved in the United States between 1985 and 2004, involving 75,873 patients (9). Increased seizure incidence was observed with antipsychotics (accounted for by clozapine and olanzapine) and drugs to treat obsessive-compulsive disorder (accounted for by clomipramine). Other drugs associated with a higher seizure incidence included alprazolam, bupropion immediate-release form, and quetiapine. Notably, the incidence of seizures was significantly lower among patients assigned to antidepressants compared with placebo (standardized incidence ratio, 0.48). In patients assigned to placebo, seizure incidence was greater than the published incidence of unprovoked seizures in community nonpatient samples, consistent with other studies showing that depressed patients have a higher incidence of seizures and epilepsy (10).

A newer class of antidepressants, serotonin-norepinephrine (NE) reuptake inhibitors (SNRIs), include the commonly prescribed venlafaxine and duloxetine. These medications increase serotonin and, to a lesser extent, norepinephrine (NE) concentrations in the brain. Thus far, they have not been examined for potential antiepileptic effects, but both proconvulsant and anticonvulsant properties may be possible depending on the dose administered (11). While there are conflicting data about seizures and NE concentrations in the cerebral cortex, many animal studies do indicate an antiepileptic effect for NE. Moreover, temporal lobe tissue removed from patients with medically refractory epilepsy during epilepsy surgery reveals depleted NE concentrations (12). While clinically important antiepileptic effects are not yet proven for SNRIs, clinical experience and reviews of published case reports indicate a significant anticonvulsant effect, with the exception of large overdoses.

The medication milnacipran can potentiate the anticonvulsant effects of conventional AEDs in a mouse model (13). The effect may be mediated through a direct action of the drug and not due to an interaction on AED concentrations. Further studies are needed to determine whether milnacipran will be useful for people with epilepsy.

ACETAZOLAMIDE

Acetazolamide (ACZ) is a carbonic anhydrase inhibitor that is active in renal, ocular, and brain tissue. Since carbonic anhydrase catalyzes the rapid interconversion of carbon dioxide and water into bicarbonate (HCO_3^-) and protons, inhibition of this enzyme prevents bicarbonate resorption in the kidneys and lowers serum pH. Carbonic anhydrase inhibitors are mainly used to treat glaucoma, altitude sickness, and benign intracranial hypertension; ACZ has been used to treat epilepsy. While ACZ does not possess any classically known antiepileptic mechanism of action, it has been used for many decades for its antiepileptic potential. Although ACZ is FDA-approved for absence epilepsy, its primary uses have been for catamenial epilepsy (see Chapter 8) and juvenile myoclonic epilepsy (14). Acetazolamide is a safe drug; however, mild paresthesia is common, kidney stones occur in approximately 1% of patients, and rare idiosyncratic reactions can occur. The risk of kidney stones is increased by dehydration and genetic factors, and it may be higher when taking other AEDs medications with carbonic anhydrase–inhibiting potential, like zonisamide and topiramate.

Acetazolamide may be prescribed daily but is often given intermittently around ovulation or perimenstrually for women with catamenial epilepsy. While the drug has never been studied in a randomized or controlled study, a telephone survey assessed women treated with ACZ for catamenial epilepsy and found that 40% believed that the drug had reduced seizures by 50% or more. However, an additional 15% of the women reported tolerance and diminished effectiveness of the drug over time. Additionally, several members of a family with an autosomal-dominant frontal lobe epilepsy achieved improved seizure control after the addition of ACZ to their AED regimen (15). Excellent control allowed AEDs to be replaced by ACZ in a few of the patients.

Interestingly, the AEDs zonisamide and topiramate also have carbonic anhydrase–inhibiting effects like ACZ. It is possible that their antiepileptic efficacy may, in part, be attributable to this mechanism.

HORMONAL THERAPY

Hormonal therapies have been used for women to alleviate seizures that occur with increased frequency perimenstrually or at other times during the menstrual cycle. Although complex and not completely understood, in general, estrogens may facilitate seizures, whereas progesterone inhibits seizures. Seizures may be more likely to occur during the menstrual cycle when progesterone levels are low and estrogens peak or in women with an inadequate luteal phase associated with abnormally low progesterone levels.

In women with partial seizures, intravenous infusion of progesterone, mimicking the luteal phase, suppresses interictal epileptiform discharges. While both progesterones and antiestrogens have been used to improve catamenial epilepsy, failure to prove long-term efficacy, irregularities in the menstrual cycle and side effects have limited the use of hormonal therapies. See Chapter 10 for a more complete discussion of this topic.

CORTICOSTEROIDS AND IMMUNOMODULATORY THERAPIES

For decades, children with West syndrome, characterized by infantile spasms and developmental delay with a highly abnormal electroencephalogram (high voltage, chaotic slowing, and multifocal spike discharges known as hypsarrhythmia), have had seizures successfully treated with adrenocorticotropic hormones (ACTH) or corticosteroids. Despite this success, corticosteroids are not standard antiepileptic therapy for most older children, adolescents, and adults with epilepsy. This is in part because there is no evidence for an immune-mediated process in most epilepsies, but it is also because trials of long-term corticosteroids may cause considerable toxicity in patients who do not have an age-dependent process like West syndrome. As a result, long-term randomized studies are not available. Toxic effects of corticosteroids include hyperglycemia, hypertension, electrolyte imbalance, cataracts, impaired wound healing, increased susceptibility to infection, osteoporosis, and suppression of the hypothalamic-pituitary-adrenal axis. Therefore, it is prudent to avoid long-term use of corticosteroids whenever possible. However, when seizures are disabling and refractory to all standard therapies, a trial of corticosteroids is reasonable. One Canadian researcher added prednisone to standard AEDs for children with medically refractory epilepsy and retrospectively reported that nearly 50% became seizure-free at a follow-up period of 1 to 5 years (16). While the results are intriguing, the study was uncontrolled, and standard AEDs were still being prescribed, so it is difficult to draw definitive conclusions about the steroid response. Some investigators are using pulse steroids such as once-a-week oral steroids to treat patients with treatment-resistant epilepsy, for which there are safety and efficacy data for treatment of ulcerative colitis (17). Safety and efficacy data are not available for pulse steroids in epilepsy.

Systemic autoimmune conditions like systemic lupus erythematosus (SLE), Hashimoto thyroiditis, and celiac disease may result in central nervous system (CNS) inflammation and seizures. Corticosteroids are widely used to reduce the CNS inflammatory response and improve seizures. While systemic autoimmune disorders often begin in other organ systems before affecting the brain, there is growing recognition of immune-mediated syndromes that primarily affect the brain. Autoimmune CNS disorders may cause seizures and other neurologic disabilities (18). Several newly discovered epilepsy syndromes are associated with antibodies to cell-surface membrane proteins such as voltage-gated potassium channels, N-methyl-D-aspartate receptors, or the enzyme glutamic acid decarboxylase. Seizures in these disorders may respond to corticosteroids alone or in combination with other immunotherapies like plasmapheresis or immunoglobulin infusion. Although quite costly now, CNS antibody testing for autoimmune causes of epilepsy will likely become routine in the near future.

Finally, in patients who present with convulsive status epilepticus without a clear etiology, immunomodulation, usually with corticosteroids, is sometimes attempted when antiepileptic medications fail to control seizures (18). For nonconvulsive status epilepticus, steroid successes are less commonly reported; many children with continuous spike and wave electroencephalographic abnormalities during slow-wave sleep are treated with corticosteroids (19–20).

CALCIUM CHANNEL BLOCKERS

Calcium channel–blocking agents (CCBs) are prescribed frequently by physicians to control heart rate and blood pressure and prevent vasospasm in patients with cardiovascular disorders. However, animal studies of CCBs also indicate anticonvulsant potential (21). While no large-scale studies of CCBs exist for the treatment of epilepsy, anecdotal reports suggest a synergistic effect when combined with traditional AEDs. Two children with severe myoclonic epilepsy of infancy had a dramatic reduction in seizure activity when verapamil was added to their AED regimen (22). One patient in status epilepticus and another with severe uncontrollable seizures were also said to benefit from verapamil (23–24). However, the mechanism for CCB effect was attributed to increased brain concentrations of AEDs due to an interaction with CCB. Substance p-glycoprotein may aid in transport of AEDs out of brain tissue. Verapamil inhibits this process, thereby increasing brain concentrations of AEDs (25). Whether the positive effects of CCBs on seizures are a direct result of their anticonvulsant properties or occur indirectly by enhancing brain AED concentrations warrants further investigation. However, a recent investigation in a canine pharmacoresistant model of epilepsy found that add-on verapamil therapy negatively impacted seizure control, which suggests that benefits may not occur in all epilepsy types (26).

CARDIAC ANTIARRHYTHMICS

Cardiac antiarrhythmic agents (CAs) are potent drugs used to control life-threatening atrial and ventricular arrhythmias. Many of the CAs, like procainamide and lidocaine, block sodium channels, similar to the effects of AEDs, such as phenytoin and carbamazepine. Despite this attribute, CAs have not been studied extensively for AED effects because they have significant toxicities, including headache, ataxia, and delirium. The narrow therapeutic window of CAs limits their utility for neurologic patients. Additionally, the use of CAs requires close surveillance and monitoring, owing to potential proarrhythmic cardiac effects. As a result, CA use has been largely confined to controlling status epilepticus in intensive care settings or to patients with severe medically refractory seizures.

The CA lidocaine was used subcutaneously to control seizures in a 10-year-old with refractory frontal lobe seizures (27). In a separate study, intravenous lidocaine was administered to 10 people with intractable epilepsy (28). In 5 of these patients, seizures ceased immediately, while 4 others had reduced frequency. Unfortunately, 4 patients experienced significant side effects that included muscle hypotonia, visual and auditory hallucinations, and bradycardia. Toxicities occurred despite therapeutic-range blood levels of the drug.

The CA mexiletine controls cardiac arrhythmias by blocking sodium channels and shortening the repolarization phase of myocardial cells. Mexiletine is effective in mice against convulsive seizures induced by electroshock and pentylenetetrazol (29). Limited data exist for human use, although one infant who did not respond to AEDs had improved seizure control (30). Mexiletine was also used to sustain the beneficial effect of lidocaine on seizures in one child with Lennox-Gastaut syndrome (31).

The potent CA amiodarone may also have antiepileptic potential. In a study of pentylenetetrazole-induced seizures, amiodarone demonstrated anticonvulsant properties (32). No clinical studies exist, most likely owing to the significant toxicities of this drug, which include lung and liver injury.

ADENOSINE

In addition to its role in energy transfer as a component of the adenosine triphosphate molecule, adenosine is a potent endogenous neuronal inhibitory neurotransmitter. The stimulatory effects of caffeine are due, in part, to its competitive inhibition with the sedating effects of adenosine. Clinically, adenosine has been used to treat supraventricular tachycardia. However, local dysfunction of the brain's adenosine may play a significant role in seizure generation (33). Unfortunately, systemic use of the drug is associated with cardiac rhythm disturbances as well as intolerable side effects that include flushing, sweating, numbness, and a feeling of impending doom. As a result, new strategies to exploit the antiepileptic potential of adenosine involve the local augmentation of adenosine through direct implantation or delivery of the compound to epileptic tissue (34). In a rat epilepsy model, adenosine was delivered locally through depth electrodes inserted into the hippocampi, and it was found that this significantly reduced seizure activity (35). Human studies have not yet been carried out.

HOMEOPATHIC MEDICINES

Homeopathy is based on the concept that substances capable of causing physical or psychological disorders can be used to remedy similar illnesses (36). Homeopaths point out that medicines are not considered homeopathic based on their diluted strengths but because of the similarity of their toxic effect to the symptoms of the disorder. Small doses of the pathogenic substance are thought to stimulate the body's own healing mechanisms against the homeopathic agent and also the underlying disorder. Homeopathy was beneficial in controlled studies of children with otitis media and in children with chemotherapy-induced stomatitis (37–38). However, there are no randomized studies of homeopathic versus allopathic treatment of epilepsy. While it is difficult to advocate for homeopathic medication treatments for epilepsy without proper scientific study, homeopathic medicine's holistic approach to epilepsy, which includes lifestyle modification and risk factor analysis, may be beneficial for many patients with uncontrolled seizures.

REFERENCES

1. Mohanraj R, Brodie MJ. Outcomes in newly diagnosed localization-related epilepsies. *Seizure*. 2005;14:318–323.
2. Boylan LS, Flint LA, Labovitz DL, Jackson SC, Starner K, Devinsky O. Depression but not seizure frequency predicts quality of life in treatment-resistant epilepsy. *Neurology*. 2004;62:258–261.
3. Markowitz JC, Brown RP. Seizures with neuroleptics and antidepressants. *Gen Hosp Psychiatry*. 1987;9:135–141.
4. Haddad PM, Dursun SM. Neurological complications of psychiatric drugs: clinical features and management. *Hum Psychopharmacol*. 2008;23:15–26.
5. Leander JD. Fluoxetine, a selective serotonin-reuptake inhibitor, enhances the anticonvulsant effects of phenytoin, carbamazepine, and ameltolide (LY201116). *Epilepsia*. 1992;33:573–576.
6. Richman A, Heinrichs SC. Seizure prophylaxis in an animal model of epilepsy by dietary fluoxetine supplementation. *Epilepsy Res*. 2007;74:19–27.
7. Favale E, Rubino V, Mainardi P, Lunardi G, Albano C. Anticonvulsant effect of fluoxetine in humans. *Neurology*. 1995;45:1926–1927.
8. Gross A, Devinsky O, Westbrook LE, Wharton AH, Alper K. Psychotropic medication use in patients with epilepsy: effect on seizure frequency. *J Neuropsychiatry Clin Neurosci*. 2000;12:458–464.
9. Alper K, Schwartz KA, Kolts RL, Khan A. Seizure incidence in psychopharmacological clinical trials: an analysis of Food and Drug Administration (FDA) summary basis of approval reports. *Biol Psychiatry*. 2007;62:345–354.
10. Kanner AM. Depression in epilepsy: a complex relation with unexpected consequences. *Curr Opin Neurol*. 2008;21:190–194.
11. Jobe PC, Browning RA. The serotonergic and noradrenergic effects of antidepressant drugs are anticonvulsant, not proconvulsant. *Epilepsy Behav*. 2005;7:602–619.
12. Pacia SV, Doyle WK, Broderick PA. Biogenic amines in the human neocortex in patients with neocortical and mesial temporal lobe epilepsy: identification with in situ microvoltammetry. *Brain Res*. 2001;899:106–111.
13. Borowicz KK, Furmanek-Karwowska K, Morawska M, Luszcki JJ, Czuczwar SJ. Effect of acute and chronic treatment with milnacipran potentiates the anticonvulsant activity of conventional antiepileptic drugs in the maximal electroshock-induced seizures in mice. *Psychopharmacology (Berl)*. 2010;207:661–669.
14. Resor SR Jr, Resor LD. Chronic acetazolamide monotherapy in the treatment of juvenile myoclonic epilepsy. *Neurology*. 1990;49:1677–1681.
15. Varadkar S, Duncan JS, Cross JH. Acetazolamide and autosomal dominant nocturnal frontal lobe epilepsy. *Epilepsia*. 2003;44:986–987.
16. Sinclair DB. Prednisone therapy in pediatric epilepsy. *Pediatr Neurol*. 28:194–198.
17. Nagata S, Shimizu T, Kudo T, et al. Efficacy and safety of pulse steroid therapy in Japanese pediatric patients with ulcerative colitis: a survey of the Japanese Society for Pediatric Inflammatory Bowel Disease. *Digestion*. 2010;81:188–192.

18. Vincent A, Irani SR, Lang B. The growing recognition of immunotherapy-responsive seizure disorders with autoantibodies to specific neuronal proteins.

19. Buzatu M, Bulteau C, Altuzarra C, Dulac O, Van Bogaert P. Corticosteroids as treatment of epileptic syndromes with continuous spike waves during slow-wave sleep. *Epilepsia.* 2009;50:68–72.

20. Okuyaz C, Aydin K, Gücüyener K, Serdaroğlu A. Treatment of electrical status epilepticus during slow-wave sleep with high-dose corticosteroid. *Pediatr Neurol.* 2005;32:64–67.

21. Luszczki JJ, Trojnar MK, Trojnar MP, Kimber-Trojnar Z, Szostakiewicz B, Zadrozniak A. Effects of amlodipine, diltiazem, and verapamil on the anticonvulsant action of topiramate against maximal electroshock-induced seizures in mice. *Can J Physiol Pharmacol.* 2008;86:113–121.

22. Iannetti P, Parisi P, Spalice A, Ruggieri M, Zara F. Addition of verapamil in the treatment of severe myoclonic epilepsy in infancy. *Epilepsy Res.* 2009;85:89–95.

23. Schmitt FC, Dehnicke C, Merschhemke M, Meencke HJ. Verapamil attenuates the malignant treatment course in recurrent status epilepticus. *Epilepsy Behav.* 2010;17:565–568.

24. Iannetti P, Spalice A, Parisi P. Calcium-channel blocker verapamil administration in prolonged and refractory status epilepticus. *Epilepsia.* 2005;46:967–969.

25. Summers MA, Moore JL, McAuley JW. Use of verapamil as a potential P-glycoprotein inhibitor in a patient with refractory epilepsy. *Ann Pharmacother.* 2004;38:1631–1634.

26. Jambroszyk M, Tipold A, Potschka H. Add-on treatment with verapamil in pharmacoresistant canine epilepsy. *Epilepsia.* 2011;52:284–291.

27. Mori K, Ito H, Toda Y, et al. Successful management of intractable epilepsy with lidocaine tapes and continuous subcutaneous lidocaine infusion. *Epilepsia.* 2004;45:1287–1290.

28. Sata Y, Aihara M, Hatakeyama K, et al. Efficacy and side effects of lidocaine by intravenous drip infusion in children with intractable seizures. *No To Hattatsu.* 1997;29:39–44.

29. Alexander GJ, Kopeloff LM, Alexander RB, Chatterjie N. Mexiletine: biphasic action on convulsive seizures in rodents. *Neurobehav Toxicol Teratol.* 1986;8:231–235.

30. Kohyama J, Shimohira M, Watanabe S, Fukuda C, Iwakawa Y. Mexiletine hydrochloride in an infant with intractable epilepsy. *Brain Dev.* 1988;10:258–260.

31. Miyamoto A, Takahashi S, Oki J. A successful treatment with intravenous lidocaine followed by oral mexiletine in a patient with Lennox-Gastaut syndrome. *No To Hattatsu.* 1999;31:459–464.

32. Ozbakis-Dengiz G, Bakirci A. Anticonvulsant and hypnotic effects of amiodarone. *J Zhejiant Univ Sci B.* 2009;10:317–322.

33. Boison D, Stewart KA. Therapeutic epilepsy research: from pharmacological rationale to focal adenosine augmentation. *Biochem Pharmacol.* 2009;78:1428–1437.

34. Boison D. Adenosine augmentation therapies (AATs) for epilepsy: prospect of cell and gene therapies. *Epilepsy Res.* 2009;85:131–141.

35. Van Dycke A, Raedt R, Dauwe I, et al. Continuous local intrahippocampal delivery of adenosine reduces seizure frequency in rats with spontaneous seizures. *Epilepsia.* 2010;51:1721–1728.

36. Taffler S. Homeopathy. In: Devinsky O, Schachter S, Pacia S, eds. *Complementary and Alternative Therapies for Epilepsy.* New York, NY: Demos Medical Publishing; 2005: 157–163.

37. Jacobs J, Springer DA, Crothers D. Homeopathic treatment of acute otitis media in children: a preliminary randomized placebo-controlled trial. *Pediatr Infect Dis J.* 2001;20: 177–183.

38. Oberbaum M, Yaniv I, Ben-Gal Y, et al. A randomized, controlled clinical trial of the homeopathic medication Traumeel S in the treatment of chemotherapy-induced stomatitis in children undergoing stem cell transplantation. *Cancer.* 2001;92:684–690.

5

Physical Treatments

The disciplines of osteopathy and its divisions of craniosacral therapy, chiropractic therapy, and massage are used to treat a diverse group of musculoskeletal disorders. Grooming, a mammalian precursor of massage, assumes an important social behavior among primates. There are strong correlates among the size of the primate neocortex, social group size, and time devoted to grooming. Among our primate ancestors, grooming may be the most widespread and effectively used method to reduce anxiety. Grooming and massage were probably the original human manual therapies. In both phylogeny and ontogeny, touch is our first sensation. Touch holds a special therapeutic power that is increasingly overlooked by the advances of Western medicine.

With the exception of skull injuries affecting the brain, there is no evidence that disorders of bones, muscles, ligaments, tendons, or other soft tissues directly cause epilepsy. However, musculoskeletal disorders can cause pain, increase stress, and reduce sleep—this may lower the seizure threshold in some individuals. Thus, there is a potential role for osteopathy, craniosacral therapy, chiropractic, and massage to reduce pain and stress, improve sleep, and secondarily increase the seizure threshold. These benefits would not be specific to the manual therapies. For example, acetaminophen and ibuprofen reduce pain; meditation and exercise can reduce stress; and sleep hygiene can improve restorative sleep. However, for some disorders, such as cervical radiculopathy, certain manual therapies may be more effective than medication.

There is no evidence that any manual therapy directly improves seizure control. Further, there is no established theoretical basis that manual therapies reduce seizure activity. Postulated mechanisms lack scientific or evidentiary support. These include improving the craniosacral (primary respiratory) rhythm and increasing blood flow to the brain. Given the lack of both strong clinical observations and a theoretical basis, it is difficult to endorse any of these therapies for epilepsy unless musculoskeletal problems are present and cause significant pain, stress, or sleep deprivation.

This chapter also includes another physical treatment, transcranial magnetic stimulation (TMS), which is being explored in epilepsy and other brain disorders. Transcranial magnetic stimulation differs from the other manual therapies as it evolved from a diagnostic tool into a potential therapy. Because repetitive TMS (rTMS) can induce long-lasting changes in the physiology of neurons, there is a theoretical basis for its potential antiseizure effect. However, data are preliminary and mixed on its potential role in treating epilepsy.

OSTEOPATHY

Osteopathic medicine (osteopathy) focuses on the musculoskeletal system to promote health and treat disease. The American Army Surgeon Andrew Still founded osteopathy in 1892. After serving in the Civil War and losing many of his children to infections, he formulated a new approach to understanding and treating medical disorders. His ideas spread to Europe and beyond. Osteopathy, like chiropractic, is a hybrid that bridges mainstream and complementary medicines. Osteopathic medicine emphasizes a holistic approach that applies a spectrum of manual and physical treatments. The 4 tenets of osteopathy are: (a) the body is an integrated unit of mind, body, and spirit; (b) the body possesses self-regulatory mechanisms, including the ability to defend, repair, and remodel itself; (c) structure and function are reciprocally related; and (d) therapy is based on these 3 principles.

Therapy most often targets musculoskeletal problems such as back and neck pain since osteopathic discipline teaches that the manipulation of bones, muscles, and joints can promote the recuperation and healing. Osteopathic manipulation differs from chiropractic manipulation in that the former is more concerned with mobilization, a procedure that moves a joint within a patient's passive range of motion.

In the United States, doctors of osteopathic medicine (DOs) are educated differently than nonphysician osteopaths. Doctors of osteopathic medicine in the United States practice as licensed physicians. They often train in the same internship and residency programs as medical doctors. Thus, many DOs practice neurology, care for people with epilepsy, and use antiepileptic drugs and other standard medical therapies. By contrast, some osteopaths—both physician and nonphysician—care for people with epilepsy using primarily physical techniques such as craniosacral therapy.

CRANIOSACRAL THERAPY

Craniosacral therapy is based on the teachings of William Sutherland (1873–1954), an American osteopathic physician who first used this manual therapy. He was struck by the resemblance between temporal and parietal bone sutures and fish gills and suggested that the cranial sutures might support a respiratory mechanism. He later claimed to have identified a rhythmic shape change in the cranial bones linked to an opposing force in the dural membranes: the reciprocal tension membrane system. The reciprocal tension membrane system is the cranium's cyclic movement of inhalation and exhalation, known as primary respiration. For Sutherland, this rhythm is vital for health and, when disrupted, it causes disease. No scientific studies can identify this rhythm using objective measures. Further, when trained craniosacral practitioners simultaneously feel for the rhythm on the same individual's skull, they report different rhythms (1–2).

In the late 1970s, John Upledger, DO, popularized craniosacral therapy, identifying what he claimed was a dural rhythm. Working with Ernest Retzlaff, Upledger reported rhythmic movements of the cranial bone (3–5). These studies did not find proof that cranial bones move or that this therapy is effective (6). There is no scientific support for major elements underlying the theoretical mechanisms of craniosacral therapy (2).

Craniosacral therapy is now widely practiced and usually involves gentle physical manipulation of the spine, skull, and cranial sutures and related soft tissues. The following premises underlie current practice: (a) the brain makes rhythmic movements at 10 to 14 cycles per minute, a frequency unrelated to the cardiac or respiratory rates; (b) small cranial pulsations can be felt with the fingertips; (c) blockages or disruptions in the normal flow of cerebrospinal fluid commonly cause symptoms and disorders; and (d) tapping the skull with fingertips can free these interferences and restore normal flow and health to bodily tissues. The "tap" is a solid, sharp, but nonpainful, blow to the head. The main goals of therapy are to open nerve passages that may be restricted, optimize the movement of cerebrospinal fluid through the spinal cord, and align bones into their healthy position. A minimal amount of force is typically applied for 30 to 180 seconds and targets multiple soft tissue structures to enlist the body's self-correcting processes. Individual sessions typically last 45 to 60 minutes. For most indications, 3 to 6 treatment sessions are completed. Depending on the disorder, subsequent maintenance sessions are done less frequently. Craniosacral therapy is used to treat many disorders, including neck and back pain, stress, temporomandibular joint syndrome, migraines, fibromyalgia, and other pain syndromes.

CHIROPRACTIC THERAPY

Chiropractic is the third largest health profession in North America behind medicine and dentistry (7). Chiropractic is intermediate between traditional and complementary alternative therapies: it does not involve drugs or surgery to prevent or treat health problems, yet it is considered by many to be mainstream and well established. Controlled studies provide limited support for the efficacy of chiropractic therapy in neck and low back pain and other disorders (as discussed later in this chapter). However, this is not true for epilepsy.

Chiropractic was founded in the 1890s by the magnetic healer D.D. Palmer in Iowa. Notably, many physicians and healers of the time used magnets, although chiropractic therapy did not. Treating a lump on the back of a man with a spinal manipulation was associated with a dramatic improvement in his hearing, as Palmer postulated it would, and chiropractic medicine was born.

The core of chiropractic therapy is manual manipulation of the spine, joints, and soft tissues. A central tenet of chiropractic is that vertebral subluxation and other disorders of spinal joints interfere with the bodily functions. Manipulation or adjustment of the spine is usually performed with high-velocity, low-amplitude thrusts delivered onto a specific spinal structure to realign or correct its abnormal position and function (i.e., subluxation). The manipulation may cause a popping or cracking sound, presumably from the gas escaping from the joint space. Within the chiropractic community, there are 2 broad views of how far the effects of spinal manipulation extend. One group holds modest claims that spinal manipulative therapy (SMT) enhances joint mobility and improves musculoskeletal symptoms. Another group believes that SMT can also improve epilepsy and other nonmusculoskeletal disorders (8–11).

Many chiropractic practitioners combine traditional techniques of spinal manipulation with mainstream medical views as well as with counseling regarding exercise, rehabilitation, ergonomics, nutrition, and lifestyle changes. In addition, other manual and alternative therapies such as acupuncture may be recommended. The strong historical opposition of chiropractic to vaccination has divided chiropractic and medical communities. Traditional chiropractic theory holds that germs do not cause disease. Although many chiropractors support vaccination, a vocal subset continues to believe that vaccines cause harm without benefit, which fosters lay fears.

The efficacy of chiropractic therapy remains hotly debated. For years, the American Medical Association (AMA) considered chiropractic an "unscientific cult," and it was a violation of AMA *Principles of Medical Ethics* for a physician to refer patients to a chiropractor. In 1987, the AMA lost an antitrust case against chiropractic, which suggests that the AMA's unfriendly posture may actually reflect fear of competition as much as a lack of scientific data and opposition to vaccines. Notably, many traditional medical practices are not supported by scientific data. However, the AMA does not typically endorse medical therapies that are not supported by controlled trials. Rigorous double-blind therapeutic trials of chiropractic are few, and the results are often inconclusive. Critical reviews of spinal manipulation therapy by chiropractors find statistically significant benefits for acute and chronic neck and low back pain, tension and migraine headaches, fibromyalgia, and cervical vertigo (12–20). In contrast, other systematic reviews by chiropractors and physicians fail to find evidence that definitely supports or refutes chiropractic efficacy for these disorders (21–25).

Complications of SMT vary from transient local discomfort, which can affect more than a third of patients, to very rare but serious complications such as arterial dissection and stroke, vertebral disc extrusion, cauda equina syndrome, myelopathy, and epidural hematoma (26). In large reviews of published studies, the frequency of adverse events varied between 33% and 60.9%, and serious adverse events ranged from 1 stroke per 20,000 manipulations to 1.46 serious adverse events per 10,000,000 manipulations and 2.68 deaths per 10,000,000 manipulations (27). No definite risk factors are known, but the use of rotatory cervical manipulation may increase the risk of stroke (28).

Chiropractic is used to treat epilepsy, but available evidence does not support its efficacy. Remarkably, one survey in the midwestern United States found that 24% of patients sought chiropractic care for their epilepsy (29). Many were likely patients with treatment-resistant epilepsy. Elsewhere, rates for chiropractic care for refractory epilepsy are likely much lower. During the past 50 years, isolated reports note that chiropractic therapy improved or "cured" epilepsy in individual cases (8, 30–33). Pistolese (8) identified 17 such case reports between 1966 and 2001. Upper cervical adjustments were used in 15 patients to correct vertebral subluxations (joint dysfunction); positive outcomes were reported in all patients. Many patients had epilepsy beginning in childhood, and 10 had a recent history of trauma. Most were treated with multiple AEDs that failed to control seizures. In many patients who improved, there was a progressive decline in the seizure frequency and duration rather than a sudden cessation of seizures after a single SMT. Several chiropractors reported that patients often required fewer AEDs after treatment began, and some patients came off AEDs.

Two illustrative cases with dramatic improvements are described. A 5-year-old boy with cerebral palsy and cortical blindness had 30 or more absence and tonic-clonic seizures per day despite therapy with phenytoin and phenobarbital (30). After 2 upper cervical adjustments during the first week, seizures declined to 10 per day. By week 3, all tonic-clonic seizures stopped, and by week 12, all seizures stopped. Over time, the neurologist withdrew all medications, and the child remained seizure-free. A 21-year-old woman with tonic-clonic and milder seizures experienced traumatic low back pain (30). She had a seizure every 3 hours lasting for 10 seconds to 30 minutes. She was referred for SMT and, during a seizure, received a cervical adjustment that abruptly stopped the seizure. At follow-up 18-months later, the patient reported that her low back complaint had resolved and her seizures had reduced in frequency to as little as 1 every 2 months.

These cases exemplify the challenge of anecdotal observations. It is impossible to refute them. For the 5-year-old boy described above, the story strongly suggests that the cervical SMT improved seizures. Most children with cerebral palsy, cortical blindness, and frequent seizures on 2 antiepileptic drugs do not have a spontaneous remission of their seizures. It is possible that their conditions were not diagnosed correctly; it is possible that their seizures improved and resolved and that the SMT was coincidental; it is possible that the SMT was therapeutic. There are other possibilities as well. This is an extremely rare observation. The 21-year-old woman is a much less convincing story. Seizures are brief, and hers could last only 10 seconds. Therefore, simply touching her for a moment could be coincidentally associated with the abrupt cessation of a seizure. However, the history is very unusual for epileptic seizures but strongly suggestive of psychogenic nonepileptic seizures. It is exceedingly rare for people with epilepsy to have seizures that routinely range in duration from 10 seconds to 30 minutes. It is also very rare for seizures to occur once every 3 hours.

Some patients with psychogenic nonepileptic seizures may be drawn to seek alternative therapies, especially if they do not accept the diagnosis and if antiepileptic drugs are ineffective. This phenomenon was observed with seizure-alert dogs: one epileptologist found that 4 of 6 patients with seizure-alert dogs had psychogenic nonepileptic seizures on video electroencephalographic monitoring (34). None of the cases reported above has data that exclude the possibility of the following: (a) nonepileptic seizures rather than epileptic seizures; (b) placebo effect; (c) coincidence with another therapeutic effect; (d) removal of an exacerbating factor; or (e) some combination of these factors.

Further, we lack any explanation why chiropractic therapy would reduce seizure activity. Several speculative suggestions include the following: (a) improved cerebral blood flow since the vertebral arteries pass through foramina in the transverse processes of the upper 6 cervical vertebrae; (b) facilitation of brain activity by correcting spinal disorders; (c) correction of abnormal biomechanics in the cervical spine that send aberrant signals from mechanoreceptors and cervical sympathetic ganglia to the brain; and (d) restoration of "hibernating" neurons back to fully functional cells through SMT (30, 35). Remember, throughout medical history, effective therapies were discovered (e.g., aspirin) before their mechanism was understood. However, this is where double-blind, randomized trials are invaluable: they define effectiveness. For chiropractic care of people with epilepsy, we lack both evidence of efficacy and a theory for why it might work.

MASSAGE

Massage is a manual technique that manipulates the superficial layers of muscle and connective tissue to promote relaxation and well being, enhance function, and relieve pain. Massage can target skin, muscles, tendons, ligaments, joints, or other connective tissue, as well as lymphatic vessels and some regions of the gastrointestinal tract. Massage can be performed with the hands, fingers, elbows, forearm, knee, or feet, or with mechanical aids. Pressure is applied with techniques that vary in intensity, focus (e.g., acupressure), movement, and sequence, and it can be combined with vibration, heat, oil, and other factors. Massage can be performed by 1 individual or 2 (synchronized) individuals. Aromatic oils, commonly used during massage, are claimed to improve seizure control in some patients (36). One study examined the effects of aromatic oils alone, aromatic oils with hypnosis, or hypnosis alone. The combination of aromatherapy with hypnosis was most effective. It would be valuable to study the efficacy of aromatherapy combined with massage in people with epilepsy in comparison with some "placebo" therapy (e.g., a nontherapeutic massage combined with perfumed oils that are not considered therapeutic) or active therapy (e.g., increased dose of an antiepileptic drug).

Massage has not been systematically studied in treating people with epilepsy. One German therapist, Bernard Müller (37), advocates therapeutic massage for epilepsy. He reported that among 361 classical acupoints, 40% were recommended or successfully used in epilepsy treatment. Compared with acupunctures with needles, the manual stimulation of acupressure allows for the potential to apply a specific manipulation during a seizure. However, there are only a few anecdotal cases where massage was helpful, and no blinded or controlled studies exist to support the benefit of massage in epilepsy. The relaxing and stress-relieving effects of massage may help some people with epilepsy since stress is often self-reported to provoke seizure activity (38).

TRANSCRANIAL MAGNETIC STIMULATION

Transcranial magnetic stimulation is a noninvasive method that uses electromagnetic induction to produce weak electric currents. It is the simplest and least invasive approach currently available to stimulate the brain. Discomfort is usually slight or absent. In TMS, a rapidly changing magnetic field located adjacent to the scalp causes the electromagnetic induction, which depolarizes neurons in the cerebral cortex. Neuronal depolarization evokes the action potential(s) that can stimulate or inhibit brain functions. When the stimulating magnet is positioned over the primary motor cortex, TMS can elicit muscle activity (motor-evoked potential). When the stimulating magnet is positioned over the occipital cortex, light flashes (phosphenes) may be experienced. In many other cortical areas, the subject is not aware of any mental or physical change, but their behavior may be slightly altered. For example, word retrieval may be impaired when language cortex is stimulated. TMS is used extensively in studies of brain function. Repetitive TMS produces longer-lasting effects that outlast the stimulation. Repetitive TMS has been assessed as a therapy for various neuropsychiatric conditions, including depression, migraines, Parkinson disease, dystonia, stroke, and tinnitus.

In epilepsy, rTMS has variable effects, but most well-controlled studies found little if any efficacy (39). In people with epilepsy, rTMS is generally well tolerated, with mild symptoms such as transient headache in approximately 10%, and seizures are very rarely activated by stimulation. The controlled study with the most positive results found that rTMS reduced seizure activity in 23 patients with malformations of cortical development (40). The benefit lasted for at least 2 months after stimulation, and there was also a reduction in interictal epileptiform discharges immediately after and 1 month after rTMS. However, a well-controlled study of 43 subjects found no benefit of rTMS over placebo in controlling seizures, but the rTMS group had a significantly lower frequency of interictal epileptiform discharges in a third of patients (41). Similarly, another study found that rTMS did not produce a significant reduction in seizure activity, but it did significantly reduce epileptiform discharges on the electroencephalogram (42). This suggests that, in some individuals, rTMS can reduce epileptiform activity. If stimulation parameters are adjusted to maximize this effect, there may be a reduction in seizure activity. One group used rTMS for 2 weeks at 0.5 Hz with a figure-eight coil placed over the seizure focus in patients with partial epilepsy (43). The number of seizures was reduced, but the frequency of interictal epileptiform discharges was unchanged.

Repetitive TMS can rarely produce seizures in patients who were seizure-free prior to stimulation or produce atypical seizures in people with epilepsy (44–46). In one review of 30 studies reporting on rTMS in people with epilepsy, only 4 patients had seizures during rTMS (1.4% of subjects). There was only 1 case of an atypical seizure that likely arose from the region of stimulation during high-frequency rTMS (46).

The jury is out on rTMS. It is safe for the vast majority of patients. Side effects are mild and transient. However, current therapeutic paradigms do not clearly provide a reduction of seizures, but data from multiple studies show that interictal epileptiform discharges can be reduced in patients with treatment-resistant epilepsy. Patients with malformations of cortical development may be particularly likely to benefit from this therapy, but replication of this finding is needed. Thus, rTMS has both a theoretical basis and support from physiology in people with epilepsy that it may be helpful. It is worth investigating more variations in treatment paradigms to identify those that may help reduce seizures.

REFERENCES

1. Green C, Martin CW, Bassett K, Kazanjian A. A systematic review of craniosacral therapy: biological plausibility, assessment reliability and clinical effectiveness. *Complement Ther Med.* 1999;7:201–207.
2. Hartman SE, Norton JM. Interexaminer reliability and cranial osteopathy. *Sci Rev Alt Med.* 2002;6:23–24.
3. Upledger JE. Craniosacral therapy. *Phys Ther.* 1995;75:328–330.
4. Upledger JE. The relationship of craniosacral examination findings in grade school children with developmental problems. *J Am Osteopath Assoc.* 1978;77:760–776.
5. Upledger JE, Karni Z. Mechano-electric patterns during craniosacral osteopathic diagnosis and treatment. *J Am Osteopath Assoc.* 1979;78:782–791.
6. Green C, Martin CW, Bassett K, Kazanjian A. A systematic review of craniosacral therapy: biological plausibility, assessment reliability and clinical effectiveness. *Complement Ther Med.* 1999;7:201–207.
7. DeVocht JW. History and overview of theories and methods of chiropractic: a counterpoint. *Clin Orthop Relat Res.* 2006;444:243–249.
8. Pistolese RA. Epilepsy and seizure disorders: a review of the literature relative to chiropractic care of children. *J Manip Physiol Ther.* 2001;24:199–205.
9. Ernst E. Chiropractic: a critical evaluation. *J Pain Symptom Manage.* 2008;35:544–562.
10. Busse JW, Morgan L, Campbell JB. Chiropractic antivaccination arguments. *J Manipulative Physiol Ther.* 2005;28:367–373.
11. Campbell JB, Busse JW, Injeyan HS. Chiropractors and vaccination: a historical perspective. *Pediatrics.* 2000;105:e43.
12. Gross A, Miller J, D'Sylva J, et al. Manipulation or mobilization for neck pain: a Cochrane Review. *Manual Ther.* 2010;4:315–333.

13. Rubinstein SM, van Middelkoop M, Assendelft WJ, de Boer MR, van Tulder MW. Spinal manipulative therapy for chronic low-back pain. *Cochrane Database Syst Rev.* 2011;2:CD008112.
14. Dagenais S, Gay RE, Tricco AC, Freeman MD, Mayer JM. NASS contemporary concepts in spine care: spinal manipulation therapy for acute low back pain. *Spine J.* 2010;10: 918–940.
15. Boline PD, Kassak K, Bronford G, Nelson C, Anderson AV. Spinal manipulation vs. amitriptyline for the treatment of chronic tension-type headaches: a randomized clinical trial. *J Manip Physiol Ther.* 1995;1:148–154.
16. Nelson CF, Bronfort G, Evans R, Boline P, Goldsmith C, Anderson AV. The efficacy of spinal manipulation, amitriptyline and the combination of both therapies for the prophylaxis of migraine headache. *J Manip Physiol Ther.* 1998;21:511–519.
17. Sarac AJ, Gur A. Complementary and alternative medical therapies in fibromyalgia. *Curr Pharm Des.* 2006;12:47–57.
18. Blunt KL, Rajwani MH, Guerriero RC. The effectiveness of chiropractic management of fibromyalgia patients. A pilot study. *J Manip Physiol Ther.* 1997;29:389–399.
19. Ernst E. Chiropractic treatment for fibromyalgia: a systematic review. *Clin Rheumatol.* 2009;28:1175–1178.
20. Nilsson N, Christensen HW, Hartvigsen J. The effects of spinal manipulation in the treatment of cervicogenic headaches. *J Manip Physiol Ther.* 1997;20:326–330.
21. Walker BF, French SD, Grant W, Green S. Combined chiropractic interventions for low-back pain. *Cochrane Database Syst Rev.* 2010;4:CD005427.
22. Gross A, Miller J, D'Sylva J, Burnie SJ, Goldsmith CH, Graham N, Haines T, Brønfort G, Hoving JL. Manipulation or mobilisation for neck pain. *Cochrane Database Syst Rev.* 2010;1:CD004249.
23. Gross A, Miller J, D'Sylva J, et al. Manipulation or mobilisation for neck pain. *Cochrane Database Syst Rev.* 2010;1:CD004249.
24. Biondi DM. Physical treatments for headache: a structured review. *Headache.* 2005;45: 738–746.
25. Astin JA, Ernst E. The effectiveness of spinal manipulation for the treatment of headache disorders: a systematic review of randomized clinical trials. *Cephalalgia.* 2002;22:617–623.
26. Senstead O, Leboueuf-Yde C, Borchgrevink C. Frequency and characteristics of side effects of spinal manipulative therapy. *Spine.* 1997;22:435–441.
27. Gouveia LO, Castanho P, Ferreira JJ. Safety of chiropractic interventions: a systematic review. *Spine.* 2009;34:E405–413.
28. Assendelft WJ, Bouter LM, Knipschild PG. Complications of spinal manipulation: a comprehensive review of the literature. *J Fam Pract.* 1996;42:475–80.
29. Liow K, Ablah E, Nguyen JC, et al. Pattern and frequency of use of complementary and alternative medicine among patients with epilepsy in the midwestern United States. *Epilepsy Behav.* 2007;10:576–582.
30. Amalu W. Cortical blindness, cerebral palsy, epilepsy and recurring otitis media: a case study in chiropractic management. *Today's Chiropractic.* 1998;27:16–25.
31. Hospers LA, Sweat RW, LaRee H, Trotta N, Seat MH. Response of a three year old epileptic child to upper cervical adjustment. *Today's Chiropractic.* 1987;15:69–76.
32. Goodman RJ, Mosby JS. Cessation of a seizure disorder: correction of the atlas subluxation complex. *J Chiropr Res Clin Invest.* 1990;6:43–46.
33. Alcantara J, Heschong R, Plaugher G, Alcantara J. Chiropractic management of a patient with subluxations, low back pain and epileptic seizures. *J Manipulative Physiol Ther.* 1998;21:410–8.
34. Krauss GL, Choi JS, Lesser RP. Pseudoseizure dogs. *Neurology.* 2007;68:308–309.

35. Gleberzon B. A chiropractic perspective on complementary and alternative therapy. In: Devinsky O, Schachter S, Pacia SV, eds. *Complementary and Alternative Therapies in Epilepsy.* New York, NY: Demos Medical Publishing; 2005:261–271.
36. Betts T. Use of aromatherapy (with or without hypnosis) in the treatment of intractable epilepsy—a two-year follow-up study. *Seizure.* 2003;12:534–538.
37. Müller B. Massage and seizure control. In: Devinsky O, Schachter S, Pacia SV, eds. *Complementary and Alternative Therapies in Epilepsy.* New York, NY: Demos Medical Publishing; 2005:65–79.
38. Mattson RH. Emotional effects on seizure occurrence. *Adv Neurol.* 1991;55:453–460.
39. Theodore WH, Fisher R. Brain stimulation for epilepsy. *Acta Neurochir Suppl.* 2007;97:261–72.
40. Fregni F, Otachi PT, Do Valle A, et al. A randomized clinical trial of repetitive transcranial magnetic stimulation in patients with refractory epilepsy. *Ann Neurol.* 2006;60:447–455.
41. Cantello R, Rossi S, Varrasi C, et al. Slow repetitive TMS for drug-resistant epilepsy: clinical and EEG findings of a placebo-controlled trial. *Epilepsia.* 2007;48:366–374.
42. Joo EY, Han SJ, Chung SH, Cho JW, Seo DW, Hong SB. Antiepileptic effects of low-frequency repetitive transcranial magnetic stimulation by different stimulation durations and locations. *Clin Neurophysiol.* 2007;118:702–708.
43. Santiago-Rodríguez E, Cárdenas-Morales L, Harmony T, Fernández-Bouzas A, Porras-Kattz E, Hernández A. Repetitive transcranial magnetic stimulation decreases the number of seizures in patients with focal neocortical epilepsy. *Seizure.* 2008;17:677–683.
44. Rosa MA, Picarelli H, Teixeira MJ, Rosa MO, Marcolin MA. Accidental seizure with repetitive transcranial magnetic stimulation. *J ECT.* 2006;22:265–266.
45. Sakkas P, Theleritis CG, Psarros C, Papadimitriou GN, Soldatos CR. Jacksonian seizure in a manic patient treated with rTMS. *World J Biol Psychiatry.* 2008;9:159–160.
46. Bae EH, Schrader LM, Machii K, et al. Safety and tolerability of repetitive transcranial magnetic stimulation in patients with epilepsy: a review of the literature. *Epilepsy Behav.* 2007;10:521–528.

6

Neurobehavioral Approaches

Many people with epilepsy (PWE) have seizures despite taking antiepileptic drugs (AEDs)or experience troubling side effects from AEDs and turn to nonpharmacologic approaches, including behavorial techniques, for help. Some PWE learn to stop their seizures using methods that they either hear about or discover for themselves. In a study of common seizure triggers and ways to stop seizures, Dahl (1) found that the most commonly used techniques by PWE to abort seizures were positive thoughts; restraining movement; and stimulation through sounds, forms of touch, or visual patterns.

Behavioral aspects of seizures have been recognized for centuries. More than 1,800 years ago, the Roman physician Galen recognized that seizures with a predictable sequence of behaviors could be stopped by stimulating an involved body part (2). The 19th-century British neurologist William Gowers (3) described how seizures could be stopped by massaging the hand where the patient felt a seizure began or by using strong aromas when a seizure started.

More recently, Dr. Peter Fenwick (4) identified the close links among brain activity, the individual's mind, and how seizures begin. He used these links as a foundation for both a behavioral model of epilepsy and the development of behavioral techniques to treat seizures (4). A scientific basis for behavioral approaches is supported by Lockard's (5) studies in which focal lesions in monkey brains involved damaged neurons surrounding the seizure focus. These cells might be influenced by thought or emotion and could therefore modulate the electrical activity in the seizure focus. Based on the modulating effect, activity in surrounding neural tissue could facilitate or inhibit seizure onset and spread. The focus of Fenwick's research is on inhibiting seizures. Given this experimental paradigm, he suggests that behavioral techniques to make the brain cells surrounding a seizure focus less likely to propagate a seizure throughout other brain structures may be a potential method to prevent seizures. Thus, teaching PWE to actively change their behaviors, thought patterns, and emotional states using various techniques tailored to the specific circumstances and events leading up to and following seizures may influence the seizure activity. Other factors that can be used to tailor the neurobehavioral approach include the location of the seizure focus, the related symptoms and emotional factors preceding seizures, and other warnings and triggers.

Changing behaviors often requires an in-depth exploration of personal, interpersonal, and lifestyle barriers. The behavioral treatment of epilepsy can help patients better understand themselves and the relationship between their seizures, their life difficulties and successes, and their relationships with others (4). It helps them reduce seizure frequency by using countermeasures to inhibit seizure activity and by avoiding seizure-prone situations. It promotes independence and better life adjustment and teaches that happiness and relaxation are powerful anticonvulsants (4).

In developing a behavioral approach to treating seizures, Fenwick (4) uses an "ABC chart" to help gather information about what leads up to a seizure and what happens during and after a seizure (4). A stands for *antecedents* (experiences that occur before and at the beginning of a seizure); B for the *behavior* that occurs during the seizure; and C for the *consequences* of the seizure. A number of neurobehavioral programs use Fenwick's ideas and this ABC chart. These programs generally address factors that contribute to a PWE's quality of life. These factors include but are not limited to seizure control; side effects of medication; mood disorders (primarily depression and anxiety, see Chapter 11); worry about seizures; social anxiety; parental/spousal anxiety; and stigma and self-mastery (the belief that a PWE can control the course of his or her life despite having epilepsy).

Two representative neurobehavioral programs that use a variety of techniques and patient-specific test results (such as electroencephalographic [EEG] findings) are discussed in this chapter along with the technique of neurofeedback and an overview of other psychosocial treatments. Readers interested in learning more are referred to the Table 6.1, a review by Mittan (6), and a book by Richards and Reiter (7).

THE ANDREWS/REITER PROGRAM

This highly structured program, devised by Donna J. Andrews, Ph.D., and Joel M. Reiter, M.D., grew out of techniques that Dr. Andrews developed to control her own complex partial seizures after medications failed. Her techniques were integrated into biofeedback methods used by Dr. Reiter to treat PWE. The goal of EEG biofeedback (discussed later in this chapter) is to teach patients to normalize their brainwave activity (recorded by an EEG) and thereby potentially reduce seizure activity (8).

A pilot study of this program and follow-up results in several countries have been encouraging (9). Individualized plans are created after first exploring patients' reasons for considering a behavioral approach and their willingness to work closely with a counselor throughout the program. The process begins by establishing a comprehensive detailed analysis of the specifics of PWE seizure onset (such as warnings in patients with partial-onset seizures, seizure symptoms, and locations of seizures) as well as the circumstances and emotional states over many

Table 6.1   Summary of Neurobehavioral Programs

Program Name	Description
FAMOSES	FAMOSES is an adaptation of the MOSES modular educational program for children with epilepsy and their parents. The goals of FAMOSES are to improve children's and their parents' knowledge about epilepsy and to help them achieve a better understanding of the disease, gain more self-confidence, and reduce specific fears regarding epilepsy. Two parallel sets of lessons are conducted for groups of 6 children and for groups of 10 parents. The child module includes orientation, basic facts, causes, diagnosis, therapy, socialization, and summary. The parent module includes overview, basic knowledge, diagnosis, therapy, prognosis, and living with epilepsy. German language.
The Penguin	The Penguin uses cartoon penguins to help children aged 3–15 years learn and talk about epilepsy in four 1.5-hour sessions. The goals of The Penguin are to guide children through their symptoms and seizures, to explain the causes of their epilepsy and their treatment, and to show them how to overcome or reduce anxiety and live as normally as possible with family and friends. These include what epilepsy is, seizure triggers, first aid, diagnostic tests, compliance, safety, and telling others. The program has been translated into English, German, Dutch, Finnish, Polish, and Hungarian.
SEE	The SEE program (formerly called Sepulveda Epilepsy Education) is a 2-day (16-hour) weekend seminar using an information medicine model that is delivered through psychoeducational techniques. The goal of the SEE program is to provide psychotherapy for people with epilepsy and their family members using an economically practical delivery system. It is the only large-audience intervention, with a typical attendance of 100–300 patients, family members, and professionals at a time. SEE is appropriate for people 12 years or older. SEE provides education about the medical aspects of epilepsy, including physiology, causes, epidemiology, diagnosis, details of medication treatment, surgery, lifestyle and triggers, first aid, and prognosis. Common problems and coping skills for the psychological and emotional challenges of epilepsy, impact on the family, effects on social functioning, and vocational adjustment are covered. SEE1 and SEE2 are 2 separate studies with different patient populations. English language.

(*continued*)

Table 6.1 Summary of Neurobehavioral Programs (*continued*)

Program Name	Description
FLIP&FLAP	FLIP&FLAP consists of 3 parallel sets of educational sessions for children older than 8 years with epilepsy, adolescents with epilepsy, and their parents. The program uses age-appropriate training materials, including cartoons and manuals. A physician and psychologist present the 2.5-day sessions. The goals are to improve (a) disease knowledge, (b) disease-related emotions, (c) communication, (d) self-responsibility, (e) self-management, (f) social participation, and {g) educational insecurity. German language.
PEPE	PEPE uses cartoons and an adult story line to teach self-care and independence to adults with epilepsy with limited intellectual functioning or other learning disabilities. The goals are to improve compliance, assist acceptance of epilepsy as a chronic illness, and support the process of becoming independent. The course consists of eight 2-hour sessions, presented by a physician and an educator, that cover common causes of epilepsy, types of seizures, treatment of epilepsy, comorbid learning and physical disabilities, prejudices, stigmatization, seizure triggers, work and employment, leisure, and social partnership. German language.
ACT program	ACT is an extension of cognitive behavior therapy. The goals are to increase psychological flexibility around the chain of seizure development, decrease the epilepsy-related experiential avoidance, broaden the person's behavior repertoire, and motivate activity in the person's chosen life direction. It involves teaching people to accept their predisposition to seize along with the fears, thoughts, and memories associated with epilepsy and to actively choose coping actions. The treatment is a combination of individual and small-group therapy aimed at seizure reduction and improved quality of life. ACT1 and ACT2 are 2 separate studies with different patient populations.
ISPE	ISPE uses the self-efficacy model of medical self-management and psychosocial coping in epilepsy. The intervention is conducted in six 2-hour sessions for 6–12 adults. Its goals are to improve self-efficacy and locus of control through goal-setting activities related to medical care and stress reduction, thereby resulting in improved quality of life. Topics include taking charge of your medical care, self-advocacy, stress, schedules and goals, relationships, and the future. English language.

Table 6.1 *(continued)*

Program Name	Description
Be Seizure Smart	Be Seizure Smart is an educational intervention for children with epilepsy and their parents via telephone. The goal is to provide individually tailored interventions for each family member by (a) providing information about epilepsy, treatment, and seizure management according to the individual's knowledge base; (b) addressing unique concerns and fears; and (c) providing emotional support. A trained nurse provides three 1-hour family sessions plus one group session with several families over a conference call. English language.
CEP	CEP consists of 2 parallel sets of four 90-minute lessons for groups of 7–10 children and adults. For the children, the goals are enhancing knowledge, self-esteem, self-care, and social communication skills; promoting responsibility on the part of the child; decreasing parental anxiety; and making it easier for both the children and their parents to live with the attendant stresses of epilepsy. For the parents, the goals are to deal with their anger, resentment, and grief related to the loss of a healthy child; increase their knowledge about caring for their child; reduce anxieties related to having a child with a seizure disorder; and improve their decision-making skills. The children's track, led by 2 professionals, includes understanding body messages, controlling seizures with medicines, telling others matter-of-factly, coping, and balancing my life. The adult track, led by one professional, consists of sharing the experience of having a child with epilepsy, making decisions and problem solving, working as a family system, and coping and adapting. Results of this single study were published in 2 separate parts: child and parent. English and Spanish language.
Ogata's program	The authors used eight 2-hour group psychotherapy sessions led by a psychologist to treat family problems among 10 adults with epilepsy. Their goal was the prevention and amelioration of family problems. Japanese language.
Gillham's program	Gillham created 2 separate one-on-one, 7-session interventions. The goal was reduction in seizure frequency and psychological symptoms. In the Self-Control of Seizures track, adults are taught how to abort seizures, control seizure triggers, and use relaxation. In the Alleviation of Psychological Disorder track, adults are counseled for a target problem individually identified for each participant. English language.

(continued)

Table 6.1 Summary of Neurobehavioral Programs (*continued*)

Program Name	Description
ACINDES	ACINDES is a small-group treatment designed for children with epilepsy and their parents. The goals are to train children to assume a leading role in the management of their health; train parents to learn to be facilitators; and train physicians to provide guidance, acting like counselors. In separate groups, children and parents (a) learn about the child's condition and to identify body signals and early warning signs; (b) recognize the elements of equilibrium and identify triggers; (c) understand treatment, therapeutic alternatives, and the usefulness of a direct patient-physician relationship; (d) handle specific risk situations (identify risks and learn strategies to handle them, including emergency home treatments); and (e) develop appropriate decision-making strategies. Spanish language.
Take Charge of Epilepsy	Take Charge of Epilepsy contains six 1-hour weekly parallel sessions for adolescents and their parents in groups of 5. The goal is to improve the quality of life of adolescents with epilepsy. Psychoeducational techniques are used to teach about adolescent issues, medical aspects, healthy lifestyle and attitudes, positive relationships with peers, family coping, stress management, and skill development. English language.

Adapted from (6).
Abbreviations: ACT, acceptance and commitment therapy; CEP, Children's epilepsy program; ISPE, intervention in self-management of people with epilepsy; MOSES, Modular Service Package Epilepsy; PEPE, Psycho Educative Programme about Epilepsy.

days leading up to seizures. Patients with seizure warnings are taught breathing techniques to institute when the warnings occur, which Andrews and Reiter (9) suggest can abort the seizure in some PWE.

Another important aspect of this program besides uncovering seizure warnings is identification of seizure triggers, which, once identified, can promote behaviors to mitigate the triggers, especially negative emotions. Patients are also taught techniques to lower stress levels and control seizures, such as deep breathing, progressive relaxation and reinforcement, and the use of biofeedback based on EEG and muscle (electromyographic) activity (10). Patients gain awareness of and learn to effectively alleviate stress-producing factors and issues in their lives, whether external or internal. In addition, they learn to communicate with others more effectively, which may decrease loneliness and isolation and increase positive feedback from others.

ACCEPTANCE AND COMMITMENT THERAPY

Acceptance and commitment therapy (ACT) is a structured behavioral therapy used for patients with depression, pain, diabetes, and other disorders (11).

Drs. Dahl and Lundgren adapted ACT to PWE and incorporated behavioral approaches in the latter stages of the ACT protocol (12).

The 6 components of ACT (13) as applied to PWE (11, 14) are introduced by a therapist to the PWE individually and as part of a group over 4 sessions. They consist of the following:

- Acceptance. People with epilepsy learn to accept aspects of epilepsy that they cannot change, including the ongoing risk of having seizures and the negative thoughts and emotions associated with the unpredictability of seizures. Patients are taught that this acceptance can paraodoxically bring better seizure control and enhance quality of life.
- *Defusion.* People with epilepsy make a distinction between themselves as people and their epilepsy, including the thoughts and feelings associated with having epilepsy. This separation allows patients to view their epilepsy objectively rather than as an integral part of the self.
- *Self as context.* Related to defusion, self as context refers to differentiating the self from life experiences, including seizures. Thus, PWE "has epilepsy but is not epilepsy." The constancy of the self is contrasted with the changing panorama of daily experiences, including seizures, which allows PWE to avoid defining themselves as epileptics, but rather to see themselves as persons with a multiplicity of life experiences, some of which are related to epilepsy.
- *Values.* People with epilepsy restore their focus on deeply held values and learn to rechannel energy toward living by and pursuing those values rather than expending energy on struggling against seizures and seizure-related issues.
- *Contact with the present moment.* People with epilepsy are taught to be fully present—to connect with the "here and now" rather than the past or the future. This "gives patients a way to let go of the struggle with their private events and to start creating the life they want" (11, p. 250).
- *Committed action.* People with epilepsy make a public commitment to focus on values and be in the present moment, while recognizing the possibility that seizures could occur.

Results in published studies, which are neither blinded nor sufficiently powered, support that ACT can reduce seizure activity and improve quality of life, with benefits sustained at 1 year follow-up (15).

NEUROFEEDBACK

Neurofeedback is a procedure that uses the EEG to help train PWE to change their brainwave patterns and reduce the likelihood of seizure occurrence, especially when seizures have not been fully controlled with tolerable doses of medication(s) (16). A technique related to neurofeedback was used successfully in experimental animal models to reduce seizures (17) and normalize EEG patterns during wakefulness and sleep (17–18).

As described by Dr. Sterman (16), who has written extensively about the use of neurofeedback for epilepsy, the first step is for a computer to comprehensively analyze brainwave rhythms while the PWE is connected to an EEG machine. While the EEG machine is still working, the PWE receives positive reinforcement on the computer screen when healthy EEG patterns are seen and negative reinforcement when EEG patterns occur that may be associated with a tendency toward seizure occurrence. Sterman's paradigm to treat epilepsy focuses on EEG operant conditioning of the sensorimotor rhythm. This sensorimotor rhythm training is arguably the best established clinical application of EEG operant conditioning. Sterman recognized that "more controlled clinical trials would be desirable," but he argued that "a respectable literature supports the clinical utility of this alternative treatment for epilepsy" (16, p. 54). The procedure that uses the skilled practice of clinical neurofeedback requires a strong background in the neurophysiologic mechanisms underlying EEG rhythms and operant learning principles and a hands-on and thorough understanding of hardware/software equipment options that the practitioner must use and individualize for the patient. Sterman's approach is to tailor the clinical practice by systematically mapping the quantitative multielectrode EEG measures in comparison with a normative database before and after treatment. These data establish the basis to guide the treatment approach and monitor progress toward EEG normalization. When effectively used, this training procedure leads to an increase in desirable EEG patterns, which may lower the probability of having seizures. Neurofeedback may also induce relaxation, though the extent to which relaxation contributes to the therapeutic benefit is unknown.

Many reports in this literature reiterate the general principles and identify small series or single pediatric or adult cases in which the factors leading to clinical improvement are uncertain since there is no control study and epilepsy is a notoriously variable disorder (19). One of the more dramatic series was reported by Walker and colleagues (20), in which the most significant abnormalities on quantitative EEG are identified, and then the EEGs in these areas are systematically "trained" back to normal. The training of EEG power was reported to reduce but rarely control seizure activity. So Walker and colleagues added coherence training to both train the power and increase the coherence. This protocol was effective in a small uncontrolled series of patients with medically refractory epilepsy. Walker and Davidson (21) replicated these positive findings in a preliminary communication on a small and uncontrolled study.

Sterman (16, 22), Walker (19–21), found neurofeedback to be safe and effective in reducing seizures in persons with drug-resistant epilepsy (16, 19–21). Some studies included a control arm in which patients received sham (and therefore presumably ineffective) neurofeedback (22).

PSYCHOSOCIAL TREATMENTS

Other psychologically based therapies and mind-body techniques have been used to reduce seizure activity in PWE (6). These methods have also been studied in children (23). Some focus on relaxation, such as yoga and meditation, and are further discussed in Chapter 13 (24–25). Others use psychological therapies, such as cognitive-behavioral therapy, that are effective in other conditions, such as depression (11). Others use education about seizures and treatment.

In reviewing these programs, Mittan (6) found that most successfully increased knowledge about epilepsy among enrollees, and some helped improve seizure control, acceptance of epilepsy, and adherence to medical treatment; increased quality of life; and improved mood and adjustment to seizures.

EVALUATING NEUROBEHAVIORAL TREATMENTS FOR EPILEPSY

Small uncontrolled or pilot studies may suggest a therapeutic effect for neurobehavioral treatments, but large, well-controlled studies are not available. Published reviews of these therapies are often critical, identifying methodological deficiencies in the studies' planning and execution (6). However, some reviews are more lenient and focus on the positive results rather than the technical limitations. Common criticisms include the following: (a) insufficient sample size limiting the power to detect significant findings; (b) lack of randomization leading to a potential selection bias; (c) lack of blinding leading to potential bias by both patient and therapist; (d) lack of a control group to provide a comparison for the natural history of the disorder, including spontaneous improvements, and to reduce the role of bias; and (e) insufficient follow-up duration to exclude short-term and potentially nonspecific treatment effects. Hence, the most recent Cochrane reviews on psychological therapies and yoga found no conclusive evidence of benefit in PWE (26–27). In addition, a recent study questions the extent to which patients can accurately identify pre-seizure warnings (28), which is an integral part of some neurobehavioral approaches.

These and other factors cast doubt about neurobehavioral therapies for many neurologists, who rely on scientific studies and objective evidence to recommend any course of treatment to PWE. However, these treatments must be individualized, so studying their effectiveness in groups of people may not be realistically possible, and ways to conclusively show whether they work for specific individual patients should be developed. This is the great catch-22 that limits the scientific study of many alternative therapies. However, without objective data, it is impossible to separate the few effective therapies from the large number of medical or alternative therapies that are either of no benefit or potentially harmful. Neurobehavioral therapies may require novel methodological approaches where patients are randomized into one therapy that is considered to be effective and another that is similar in appearance but considered ineffective based on its specific methodology. Such a study would be simple to accomplish for neurofeedback, but it has not yet been done with sufficient size and methodology. It would be harder, but not impossible, to achieve either a neurobehavioral approach to identifying seizure precipitants or modification of attitudes and strategies to prevent seizures.

CONCLUSION

Several neurobehavioral approaches to prevent or lessen the severity of seizures and improve overall quality of life for PWE have been developed. Convincing evidence for the effectiveness of these approaches is not presently available, largely as a consequence of the challenges in designing definitive research studies. However, there is general agreement that these approaches are safe. Additional research may clarify if and how they work and, if they do, who is most likely to benefit.

When possible, people with epilepsy should be empowered when possible to become active partners in managing their health, and neurobehavioral approaches can potentially play a key role in this process. Therefore, conclusively demonstrating whether PWE can avoid or terminate seizures as well as be enabled to enhance their overall quality of life through existing or new neurobehavioral approaches is an important and worthwhile goal.

REFERENCES

1. Dahl J. A behaviour medicine approach to epilepsy—time for a paradigm shift? *Scand J Behav Ther*. 1999; 28:97–114.
2. Temkin O. *The Falling Illness*. Baltimore, MD: The Johns Hopkins Press; 1945.
3. Gowers W. *Epilepsy, and Other Chronic Convulsive Diseases*. London, England: Churchill; 1881.
4. Fenwick P. Seizure generation. In: Devinsky O, Schachter S, Pacia S, eds. *Complementary and Alternative Therapies for Epilepsy*. New York, NY: Demos Medical Publishing; 2005:43–52.
5. Lockard JS. A primate model of clinical epilepsy: mechanism of action through quantification of therapeutic effects. In: Lockard JS, Ward AA, eds. *Epilepsy: A Window to Brain Mechanisms*. New York, NY: Raven Press; 1980:11–49.
6. Mittan R. Psychosocial treatment programs in epilepsy: a review. *Epilepsy Behav*. 2009;16:371–380.
7. Richards A, Reiter JM. *Epilepsy: A New Approach*. New York, NY: Walker & Co; 1995.
8. Lantz D, Sterman M. Neuropsychological assessment of subjects with uncontrolled epilepsy: effects of EEG feedback training. *Epilepsia*. 1988;29:163–171.
9. Andrews DJ, Reiter JM. In: Devinsky O, Schachter S, Pacia S, eds. *Complementary and Alternative Therapies for Epilepsy*. New York, NY: Demos Medical Publishing; 2005:33–42.
10. Reiter JM, Andrews DJ, Janis C. *Taking Control of Your Epilepsy: A Workbook for Patients and Professionals*. Santa Rosa, CA: Andrews/Reiter Epilepsy Research Program; 1987. Available from Andrews/Reiter Epilepsy Research Program, 1103 Sonoma Avenue, Santa Rosa, CA 95405.
11. Dahl JC, Lundgren TL. Conditioning mechanisms, behavior technology, and contextual behavior therapy. In: Schachter SC, Holmes GL, Trenite DGAK, eds. *Behavioral Aspects of Epilepsy: Principles & Practice*. New York, NY: Demos Medical Publishing; 2008:245–252.
12. Dahl J. *Epilepsy: A Behavior Medicine Approach to Assessment and Treatment in Children*. Göttingen, Germany: Hogref & Huber; 1992.

13. Lundgren T. A development and evaluation of an integrative health model in the treatment of epilepsy [master's thesis]. Uppsala, Sweden: University of Uppsala; 2004.
14. Dahl J, Lundgren T. Behavior analysis of epilepsy: conditioning mechanisms, behavior technology and the contribution of ACT. *Behav Anal Today*. 2005;6:191–202.
15. Lundgren T, Dahl J, Melin L, Kies B. Evaluation of acceptance and commitment therapy for drug refractory epilepsy: a randomized trial in South Africa: a pilot study. *Epilepsia*. 2006;47:2173–2179.
16. Sterman MB. Neurofeedback therapy. In: Devinsky O, Schachter S, Pacia S, eds. *Complementary and Alternative Therapies for Epilepsy*. New York, NY: Demos Medical Publishing; 2005:53–56.
17. Sterman MB. Studies of EEG biofeedback training in man and cats. In: *Highlights of the 17th Annual Conference. VA Cooperative Studies in Mental Health and Behavioral Sciences*. Washington, DC: U.S. Government; 1972:50–60.
18. Sterman MB, Howe RD, Macdonald LR. Facilitation of spindle-burst sleep by conditioning of electroencephalographic activity while awake. *Science*. 1970;167:1146–1148.
19. Walker JE, Kozlowski GP. Neurofeedback treatment of epilepsy. *Child Adolesc Psychiatr Clin N Am*. 2005;14:163–176.
20. Walker JE, Weber R, Norman C. Importance of QEEG guided coherence training for patients with mild closed head injury. *J Neurotherapy*. 2002;6:31–42.
21. Walker JE, Davidson D. Long term remediation of seizures in refractory epilepsy with QEEG-guided neurofeedback training [abstract]. Presented at the Society for Neuronal Regulation Meeting; August 21–24, 2003; Houston, TX.
22. Sterman MB, Egner T. Foundation and practice of neurofeedback. *Appl Psychophysiol Biofeedback*. 2006;31:21–35.
23. Kneen R, Appleton RE. Alternative approaches to conventional antiepileptic drugs in the management of paediatric epilepsy. *Arch Dis Child*. 2006;91:936–941.
24. Lansky EP, St. Louis EK. Transcendental meditation: a double-edged sword in epilepsy? *Epilepsy Behav*. 2006;9:394–400.
25. Yardi N. Yoga for control of epilepsy. *Seizure*. 2001;10:7–12.
26. Ramaratnam S, Baker G, Goldstein L, Ramaratnam S. Psychological treatments for epilepsy. *Cochrane Database Syst Rev*. 2005;4:CD002029.
27. Ramaratnam S, Sridharan K. Yoga for epilepsy. *Cochrane Database Syst Rev*. 2000;3: CD001524.
28. Maiwald T, Blumberg J, Timmer J, Schulze-Bonhage A. Are prodromes preictal events? A prospective PDA-based study. *Epilepsy Behav*. 2011;21:184–188.

7

Countering the Effects of Antiepileptic Drugs, Seizures, and Brain Injury

Nearly 1 in 3 people with epilepsy (PWE) continues to have seizures despite taking prescription seizure medications and antiepileptic drugs (AEDs) and experiences seizure-related physical, emotional, and social consequences (1–2). In addition, many PWE experience troubling side effects from AEDs, either within minutes or hours of taking their pills or over months to years. Still other PWE live with the daily, often constant, difficulties caused by brain injuries, such as those due to head trauma or stroke, which may have caused their epilepsy. It is therefore understandable that some PWE turn to alternative treatments, such as herbal remedies, dietary supplements, or vitamins, to improve these problems.

Presently, there are no published clinical trials in PWE of alternative therapies for the treatment of AED side effects, the after effects of seizures, or the persistent complications of brain injuries. Therefore, there is no definitive evidence of their safety, tolerability, or effectiveness in PWE. However, new approaches to the scientific study of these therapies are underway in many laboratories and medical centers, which will help to establish their risks and benefits for PWE.

This chapter discusses the alternative therapies most often taken or researched as treatments for common AED adverse effects, seizures and brain injuries, specific problems with cognition (primarily memory), migraine headaches, and effects on bone health.

COGNITION

Problems with cognition—or thinking—commonly occur after seizures for a period of time and can also result from brain injuries and AED side effects. Cognition refers to many different kinds of thinking-related functions, including memory, language, judgment, and concentration/attention. Many complementary and alternative medicine (CAM) therapies for cognitive dysfunction, especially for memory dysfunction, have been tried and studied, such as *Ginkgo biloba*, acetyl-L-carnitine, cytidine 5'-diphosphocholine (CDP-choline), and vinpocetine. Not surprisingly, since memory problems are common in PWE (3), Ekstein and Schachter (4) found that *Ginkgo biloba* was one of the most commonly taken herbal remedies by PWEs.

Ginkgo biloba is a popular herbal remedy that is extracted from the leaves of the maidenhair tree and has been used in traditional Chinese medicine for centuries for various disorders. Many studies evaluated *Ginkgo biloba* for cognitive decline or dementia, but most of these clinical trials were methodologically limited. For example, many included only small numbers of subjects and were short in duration. A comprehensive review of clinical trials concluded there was inconsistent and unreliable evidence for *Ginkgo biloba* having a clinically significant beneficial effect for dementia or cognitive impairment, although it appears to be safe (5).

Acetyl-L-carnitine is a carnitine derivative that may increase the effects of the brain neurotransmitter acetylcholine, which is vital for memory function. Blocking acetylcholine receptors in healthy subjects impairs memory. The availability of acetylcholine progressively diminishes in certain brain cells of persons with Alzheimer disease, but studies of acetyl-L-carnitine in Alzheimer disease found no benefit using objective measures of cognition, severity of dementia, or functional ability (6). Some drugs used to treat Alzheimer disease increase the amount of acetylcholine available at the synapse. These drugs show small efficacy in large (well-powered) randomized, double-blind trials for Alzheimer disease but have never been shown in similar trials to improve memory in other patient groups or healthy individuals.

Cytidine 5'-diphosphocholine is a widely available dietary supplement that is a necessary building block for the synthesis of phosphatidylcholine, an important component of cell membranes throughout the body. Cytidine 5'-diphosphocholine is an active ingredient of soy lecithin. It is prescribed in Europe for cognitive dysfunction, particularly in patients with a history of strokes. A review of published studies concluded that CDP-choline had a positive effect on memory over at least a short to medium duration and was also determined to be well tolerated (7).

Vinpocetine is derived from the leaves of the lesser periwinkle (*Vinca minor*). It has been used for decades for various conditions, especially in Eastern Europe. A review of 3 studies evaluating its safety and effectiveness for cognitive impairment showed few side effects and benefit associated with doses of 30 mg/d and 60 mg/d compared with placebo, but the number of patients treated for 6 months or more was small. This review found that the evidence that vinpocetine improves cognitive dysfunction was inconclusive (8).

Other studies of herbal remedies, foods, and vitamins have either not been replicated or yielded inconsistent findings in the treatment of cognitive dysfunction. These studies included assessments of chromium (9), blueberry juice (9), vitamin B_6 (10), folic acid and vitamin B_{12} (11), iron supplements (12), *Bacopa monniera*, and phosphatidylserine.

HEADACHE

The most common types of headaches are muscle tension and migraine headaches. People with epilepsy are about twice as likely to have migraine headaches compared with the general population (13). Similarly, persons with migraine are twice as likely to have epilepsy compared with others (14). In PWE, migraines can occur just before seizures (preictal), between seizures (interictal), during seizures (ictal), or after seizures (postictal). Interictal and postictal headaches (PIHs) are the most common.

Migraine headaches in PWE are similar to migraines in people without epilepsy. A migraine may start with vague symptoms or a change in mood/thinking for hours to even days before the headache starts; typically, these are symptoms that the individual recognizes as having preceded their migraines before. Closer to the beginning of the headache, sometimes lasting for a period of time during the headache, symptoms called the *aura* may occur. The most common type of aura is an alteration of vision, especially to one side or the other, that develops slowly over minutes and lasts less than an hour. Tingling or numbness may also occur. The headache is usually one-sided, throbbing, painful, and made worse by physical exertion as well as sensory stimulation (e.g., bright lights, loud noises, strong smells). It may last hours to up to 2 or 3 days, and nausea and vomiting often occur. When severe, the vomiting can prevent patients from taking their AEDs, and it may be useful to use either antinausea/antiemetic medications or a benzodiazepine (e.g., dissolvable clonazepam wafer) that does not need to be swallowed. Once the headache ends, other symptoms may be prominent, such as fatigue and changes in mood.

Like interictal migraines, PIHs are usually moderate to severe in intensity, last for many hours, and also have the characteristics of migraine. They can occur after partial seizures and particularly after generalized tonic-clonic seizures. Young adults with epilepsy who have a history of interictal headaches seem to be particularly vulnerable, as are persons with drug-resistant seizures (15). Postictal headaches often have a significant impact on the quality of life of PWE, sometimes more than seizures, and may be the main clue for PWE that they just had a seizure.

Most often, headaches in PWEs do not reflect any structural abnormality in the brain. Sometimes, however, headaches may be due to the same underlying condition that causes seizures in a given PWE, such as brain trauma, a tumor, or an abnormality of blood vessels in the brain called an arteriovenous malformation.

Headaches can also be side effects of AEDs. The severity of AED-related headaches usually reflects how quickly the medication is initiated and the total daily dose. Mild AED-related headaches tend to improve or resolve over time or with a dosage adjustment, but more severe headaches may persist and interfere with a person's ability to think or function.

Many prescription drugs are approved by the Food and Drug Administration for migraine headaches. Some are taken when a migraine starts with the goal of ending it (i.e., symptomatic drugs). Others are taken every day to prevent migraines from occurring (e.g., prophylactic drugs). Two such drugs—valproate and topiramate—are also approved for seizures. There are no specific treatments that are proven safe and effective for PIH other than preventing seizures from occurring. Over-the-counter pain medications such as aspirin, nonsteroidal antiinflammatory drugs, and acetaminophen can help (16). Other therapies used for migraine headaches, such as ice packs to the forehead and temple (or other affected head regions) as well as rest in a quiet, dark place, are often helpful for PWE.

Persons with chronic headaches often use herbal remedies. Wells et al (17) compared the use of CAM between adults with and without common neurologic conditions using the 2007 National Health Interview Survey of 23,393 sampled U.S. adults. Nearly half of adults with migraine headaches reported use of CAM, and about half of this group used herbal remedies or dietary supplements. A number of research studies evaluated the safety and effectiveness of CAM for migraines, but none of these studies has focused on PWE. Therefore, the benefits or risks of these treatments in PWE are unknown.

Feverfew is derived from dried chrysanthemum leaves. While some studies found that feverfew prevents migraine headaches, concerns have been raised about the quality of these and other studies, supporting the conclusion that definitive benefit remains unproven (18–19). Potential side effects include sore mouth and tongue (including ulcers), swollen lips, loss of taste, abdominal pain, and gastrointestinal disturbances (20).

Petadolex (*Petasites hybridus* [PH]) is an extract of Butterbur root. In addition to headaches, *Petasites hybridus* has been used for respiratory problems, such as asthma, and gastrointestional/urogenital tract problems (to reduce spasms). Published studies showed promising effects in preventing migraines, but based on the relatively small number of subjects studied, further research is needed to firmly establish safety and effectiveness (21–22). Side effects include temporary liver dysfunction and mild gastrointestinal disturbances.

Melatonin was studied for cluster headaches, which is related in some patients to migraine headaches. In one double-blind, placebo-controlled, clinical study of 20 patients, melatonin reduced cluster headache in 50% of treated patients (23). Studies in persons with migraine headaches or on headaches in PWE, however, are lacking.

Other research studies have produced inconsistent findings for a variety of herbal remedies, foods, and vitamins, including magnesium, green tea, megadose vitamins C and E, lipoic acid, vitamin B_2 (riboflavin), coenzyme Q10, and *Ginkgo biloba*. Nonetheless, there is growing scientific evidence to support the further study of some of these treatments in the laboratory and with patients who have migraines (24).

Finally, a comprehensive review evaluated 22 clinical trials with 4,419 participants in which acupuncture was evaluated for the acute treatment of as well as the prevention of migraines. The review concluded that acupuncture is at least as effective as, or possibly more effective than, preventative drug treatment, with fewer adverse effects. Therefore, acupuncture should be considered a treatment option for patients willing to undergo this treatment (25).

BONE HEALTH

Healthy, strong bones derive their strength and density from minerals, most importantly calcium. A bone mineral density (BMD) test measures a person's level of bone minerals, which are then compared with levels expected for persons of the same age and sex. The most accurate BMD test is the dual energy x-ray absorptiometry scan, which is painless, takes about 20 minutes, and exposes the patient to minimal radiation. A slightly lower-than-normal BMD for age and sex is referred to as osteopenia, whereas more pronounced bone mineral loss is called osteoporosis, a condition that weakens bones and significantly increases the risk of bone fractures, especially of the hip, spine, and wrist.

Osteoporosis affects millions of older Americans, women more than men. Postmenopausal women are particularly vulnerable because the ovaries stop producing estrogen at menopause, and estrogen protects bones from the loss of minerals. Other risk factors for osteoporosis include having small bones, smoking, alcohol intake, inadequate calcium or protein in the diet, lack of exercise, and genetic factors. Osteoporosis due to aging is called primary osteoporosis; when due to other causes, osteoporosis is classified as secondary.

For several reasons, PWE and especially women with epilepsy (WWE) are at increased risk for bone fractures, osteopenia, and both primary and secondary osteoporosis (26–28). Fractures can occur from falls due to seizures, such as tonic-clonic seizures, or from severe dizziness caused by seizure medications. Loss of minerals from bones can result from early menopause, which affects some WWE, and from long-term use of certain AEDs, including phenobarbital, primidone, phenytoin, carbamazepine, oxcarbazepine, and valproate, which are thought to cause secondary osteoporosis by reducing vitamin D levels (29).

The best way to treat osteopenia and osteoporosis is to prevent bone mineral loss from ever occurring with a diet high in calcium and vitamin D, and with adequate exposure to sunlight (ultraviolet light (UVB)), which converts 7-dehydrocholesterol into vitamin D3. Weight-bearing exercise increases BMD before menopause and slows bone loss after menopause. Taking over-the-counter calcium and vitamin D supplements is recommended for WWE taking AEDs that are associated with bone mineral loss. The generally accepted doses are 1,000 mg of calcium and 400 IU of vitamin D daily for premenopausal women, and 1,500 mg calcium and 600 IU vitamin D daily for postmenopausal women (30). Women with epilepsy taking phenytoin should be aware that calcium supplements may decrease blood levels of phenytoin. Notably, in recent years, the lower range of "normal" vitamin D in the blood has been revised upward. The vitamin D level in the blood can be checked on routine blood work. For WWE who take medications that accelerate the metabolism of vitamin D (e.g., phenytoin, carbamazepine, phenobarbital, primidone) or alter vitamin D in other ways (e.g., valproate), larger amounts of daily vitamin D (e.g., 2,000 IU per day) should be considered. Vitamin D is often given in the form of cholecalciferol, also called vitamin D_3. Prescription drugs that are sometimes used, especially for women diagnosed with osteoporosis, are biphosphonates and hormone replacement therapy with estrogen.

Other natural substances—onion, garlic and parsley; the essential oils of sage, rosemary, thyme, and other herbs; soya; and several herbal medicines associated with traditional Chinese and Ayurvedic medicine—have all demonstrated promising effects in animal models of osteoporosis but have not yet been studied or been proven effective in clinical studies (31).

CONCLUSION

Many complementary approaches to alleviate the side effects of AEDs and after-effects of seizures or to lessen the consequences of brain injuries have been tried by PWEs and studied in populations without epilepsy. Convincing evidence for the effectiveness of these approaches is not presently available, with the exception of CDP-choline for cognitive dysfunction associated with cerebrovascular disease and acupuncture for migraine headaches. None of these treatments have yet been suitably studied in PWE. However, there is general agreement that many of the food substances, dietary supplements, and herbal medicines used to treat cognitive dysfunction, migraine headaches, and bone loss are safe. Additional research will hopefully further clarify which, if any, of these treatments work safely for PWE and, if they do, who is most likely to benefit.

People with epilepsy who try natural products should inform their physician, since they could affect the blood levels of other medications, including AEDs. In addition, natural products might cause side effects that the physician might otherwise attribute to an AED or result in an increase of seizures, leading to an erroneous conclusion that the prescribed AED is ineffective.

REFERENCES

1. Kwan P, Brodie MJ. Early identification of refractory epilepsy. *N Engl J Med*. 2000;342: 314–319.
2. Kwan P, Arzimanoglou A, Berg AT, et al. Definition of drug resistant epilepsy: Consensus proposal by the ad hoc Task Force of the ILAE Commission on Therapeutic Strategies. *Epilepsia*. 2009;51:1069–1077.
3. LaFrance WC Jr, Kanner AM, Hermann B. Psychiatric comorbidities in epilepsy. *Int Rev Neurobiol*. 2008;83:347–383.
4. Ekstein D, Schachter SC. Natural products in epilepsy—the present situation and perspectives for the future. *Pharmaceuticals*. 2010;3:1426–1445.
5. Birks J, Grimley Evans J. *Ginkgo biloba* for cognitive impairment and dementia. *Cochrane Database Syst Rev*. 2007:CD003120.

6. Hudson S, Tabet N. Acetyl-L-carnitine for dementia. *Cochrane Database Syst Rev.* 2003:CD003158.

7. Fioravanti M, Yanagi M. Cytidinediphosphocholine (CDP-choline) for cognitive and behavioural disturbances associated with chronic cerebral disorders in the elderly. *Cochrane Database Syst Rev.* 2004:CD000269.

8. Szatmari SZ, Whitehouse PJ. Vinpocetine for cognitive impairment and dementia. *Cochrane Database Syst Rev.* 2003;CD003119.

9. Krikorian R, Eliassen JC, Boespflug EL, Nash TA, Shidler MD. Improved cognitive-cerebral function in older adults with chromium supplementation. *Nutr Neurosci.* 2010;13:116–122.

10. Malouf M, Grimley Evans J. The effect of vitamin B_6 on cognition. *Cochrane Database Syst Rev.* 2003:CD004393.

11. Malouf M, Grimley EJ, Areosa SA. Folic acid with or without vitamin B_{12} for cognition and dementia. *Cochrane Database Syst Rev.* 2003:CD004514.

12. Falkingham M, Abdelhamid A, Curtis P, Fairweather-Tait S, Dye L, Hooper L. The effects of oral iron supplementation on cognition in older children and adults: a systematic review and meta-analysis. *Nutr J.* 2010;9:4.

13. Ottman R, Lipton RB. Comorbidity of migraine and epilepsy. *Neurology.* 1994;44:2105–2110.

14. Lipton RB, Ottman R, Ehrenberg BL, Hauser WA. Comorbidity of migraine: the connection between migraine and epilepsy. *Neurology.* 1994:44:S28–S32.

15. Ekstein D, Schachter SC. Postictal headache. *Epilepsy Behav.* 2010;19:151–155.

16. Syvertsen M, Helde G, Stovner LJ, Brodtkorb E. Headaches add to the burden of epilepsy. *J Headache Pain.* 2007;8:224–230.

17. Wells RE, Philips RS, Schachter SC, McCarthy EP. Complementary and alternative medicine use among U.S. adults with common neurological conditions. *J Neurol.* 2010;257:1822–1831.

18. Pittler MH, Ernst E. Feverfew for preventing migraine. *Cochrane Database Syst Rev.* 2004:CD002286.

19. Vogler BK, Pittler BK, Ernst E. Feverfew as a preventative treatment for migraine: a systematic review. *Cephalalgia.* 1998;18:704–708.

20. Evans RW, Taylor FR. "Natural" or alternative medications for migraine prevention. *Headache.* 2006;46:1012–1018.

21. Grossman M, Schmidramsl H. An extract of *Petasites hybridus* is effective in the prophylaxis of migraine. *Int J Clin Pharmacol Ther.* 2000;38:430–435.

22. Lipton RB, Gobel H, Einhaupl KM, Wilks K, Mauskop A. *Petasites hybridus* root (butterbur) is an effective preventive treatment for migraine. *Neurology.* 2004;63:2240–2244.

23. Leone M, D'Amico D, Moschianof, Fraschini F, Bussone G. Melatonin versus placebo in the prophylaxis of cluster headache: a double-blind pilot study with parallel groups. *Cephalgia.* 1996;16:494–496.

24. Taylor FR. Nutraceuticals and headache; the biological basis. *Headache.* 2011;51:484–501.

25. Linde K, Allais G, Brinkhaus B, Manheimer E, Vickers A, White AR. Acupuncture for migraine prophylaxis. *Cochrane Database Syst Rev.* 2009:CD001218.

26. Persson HBI, Alberts KA, Farahmand BY, Tomson T. Risk of extremity fractures in adult outpatients with epilepsy. *Epilepsia.* 2002;43:768–772.

27. Souverein PD, Webb DJ, Petri H, Weil J, van Staa TP, Egberts ACG. Incidence of fractures among epilepsy patients: a population based retrospective cohort study in the General Practice Research database. *Epilepsia.* 2005;46:304–310.

28. Vestergaard P. Epilepsy, osteoporosis and fracture risk: a meta analysis. *Acta Neurol Scand.* 2005;112:277–286.

29. Vestergaard P, Rejnmark L, Mosekilde L. Fracture risk associated with use of antiepileptic drugs. *Epilepsia*. 2004;45:1130–1137.

30. Cramer JA, Gordon J, Schachter S, Devinsky O. Women with epilepsy: hormonal issues from menarche through menopause. *Epilepsy Behav*. 2007;11:160–178.

31. Putnam SE, Scutt AM, Bicknell K, Priestley CM, Williamson EM. Natural products as alternative treatments for metabolic bone disorders and for maintenance of bone health. *Phytother Res*. 2007;21:99–112.

8

Women's Issues

Epilepsy presents special issues for women. These concerns include the relationship of seizures to menstrual cycle–related hormone changes, sexuality, birth control, fertility, birth defects related to antiepileptic drugs (AEDs),
changes in AED levels and seizure susceptibility in pregnancy, and menopause. Several disorders of reproductive function occur in women with epilepsy
(Table 8.1).

Puberty includes the development of breasts, pubic hair, menstruation,
changes in body fat distribution, acne, and body odor. Sexual maturation, which
also includes neurobehavioral and psychosocial changes, begins between ages 9
and 12 years and extends over several years for most girls, with the first menstruation usually occurring between ages 10 and 14 years. The onset of puberty has
declined steadily over the past century, likely reflecting the consumption of more
calories in childhood, which are converted to fat. Sufficient fat supplies signal
the brain that resources are available to support pregnancy. Other factors may
account for the earlier onset of menarche, including a reduction in chronic infec-
tious and other illnesses, psychological stress, and possibly environmental toxins
such as bisphenol A (present in many plastic bottles).

The age of puberty overlaps with the offset and onset of several epilepsy
syndromes, but there is no clear evidence that reproductive hormones (e.g.,
testosterone, estrogen, or progesterone) are major factors in determining when
children outgrow epilepsy or when epilepsy begins. For example, many children
with childhood absence epilepsy outgrow epilepsy before, during, or after onset
of puberty. Similarly, temporal lobe epilepsy and juvenile myoclonic epilepsy can
begin before, during, or after the onset of puberty. When offset or onset occurs
around the time of puberty, it is often linked causally to puberty, but the relationship is likely coincidental in many cases. Since sex hormones bind to neuronal receptors in the brain, these hormones can influence seizure threshold,
and physiologic changes during puberty could influence the course of epilepsy
in some cases. Since estrogen and progesterone can affect the seizure threshold,
hormonal influences on epilepsy appear to be greatest in females.

Table 8.1   Disorders of Reproductive Function

Hyperandrogenism
Polycystic ovarian syndrome
Menstrual irregularities/anovulatory cycles
Infertility

THE MENSTRUAL CYCLE AND SEIZURES

Many women with epilepsy report that seizures are more frequent during—or even restricted to—certain portions of their menstrual cycle. Medical studies support this relationship, which is referred to as catamenial epilepsy. Catamenial epilepsy occurs with all seizure types, including idiopathic generalized and partial seizures. For women with catamenial epilepsy, seizures are most frequent during the premenstrual, menstrual, and ovulatory periods. Occasionally, there is an increase in seizure frequency during the entire 2 weeks before the onset of menstruation (luteal phase), extending from ovulation through the menstrual onset (1).

Catamenial seizure patterns result from changes in the total and relative concentrations of estrogen and progesterone. Estrogen has various functions in the body as well as the brain. In addition to regulating reproductive functions, it modulates neurotransmission and blood flow and has excitatory effects on neurons by enhancing N-methyl-D-aspartate–mediated glutamate receptor activity (2). Therefore, estrogen can lower the seizure threshold. In contrast, progesterone, especially its active metabolite allopregnanolone, has inhibitory effects by potentiating γ-aminobutyric acid type A–mediated chloride conductance (3). Progesterone can raise the seizure threshold. When the ratio of estrogen to progesterone rises during the premenstrual time, seizures are more likely to occur. Although both estrogen and progesterone levels decline premenstrually, there is a more dramatic decline in progesterone levels. This progesterone withdrawal appears to lower the seizure threshold during the days just before menses and on the first day of menstruation (4). By contrast, estrogen levels rise and reach a peak just before ovulation at the midcycle. This estrogen peak contributes to increased seizure susceptibility when ovulation occurs midcycle.

The luteal phase, the 2 weeks prior to menses, is also a time when some women are more likely to have seizures, especially during those months when ovulation does not occur. Women with epilepsy have more frequent menstrual cycles in which they do not ovulate (anovulatory cycle) than women without epilepsy (5). Progesterone levels are low during anovulatory cycles, fostering a hormonal milieu in which seizures are more likely to occur.

TREATMENT OF CATAMENIAL EPILEPSY

For women whose seizures are more frequent at certain times of the menstrual cycle, that time represents an especially critical period for them to adhere to their medication regimen, get good sleep, and avoid stress and excess alcohol and other factors that may provoke their seizures. No herbal product, medication, or other therapy is proven to prevent seizure exacerbations related to the menstrual cycle in randomized, blinded trials. Some reported therapies for catamenial seizure are discussed in this chapter.

PROGESTERONE

Progesterone has been used to prevent catamenial exacerbations. Progesterone is mainly usually used for obstetric and gynecologic indications to suppress the menstrual cycle or as a cyclic therapy to supplement endogenous progesterone levels during the luteal phase and then withdraw it before the menses. Progestational therapy can use either synthetic or natural agents. Synthetic progesterone, the main form used in birth control pills and in hormone replacement therapy (HRT), does not appear to be as effective in preventing seizures as natural progesterone since the synthetic form may not be active in the same brain areas (6). However, synthetic progesterone has not been adequately studied, and its efficacy remains uncertain in catamenial epilepsy.

Natural progesterone can be given in a pill (Prometrium), lozenge, or cream. To treat catamenial epilepsy, natural progesterone is usually recommended. Natural progesterone can be derived from an extract of soy or yams and is available in 25- to 200-mg doses. Since the half-life is approximately 5 hours, it is often given 3 times daily. Several pilot studies found no significant benefit from the synthetic norethisterone or medroxyprogesterone (Provera), while several open-label studies found significant reductions with natural progestins (7–10). The studies that found benefits used natural progesterone for seizure exacerbations during the 2 weeks prior to menses and ending after the first day of menstrual flow. A larger National Institutes of Health study is ongoing to assess natural progesterone in a randomized, controlled trial. Side effects are usually mild and include sedation, depressed mood, breast tenderness, and vaginal spotting.

INCREASED DOSES OF AEDS OR ADDITIONAL AEDS

When the timing of the menstrual-related exacerbation of seizures is predictable, a currently used AED drug dose can be temporarily increased, or a short-term AED can be added during the vulnerable period. If a woman takes an AED with a short- to moderate-duration half-life (e.g., 4–16 hours), the dose can be increased around the period of increased seizure susceptibility (e.g., premenstrually) and continued until this time has passed. Depending on the specific patient and AED regimen, an increase of 10% to 25% of the total daily dose of one AED for 2 to 5 days is usually well tolerated. However, some patients are very sensitive to small dose changes. Unfortunately, this strategy may fail as seizures still occur during the vulnerable period or are delayed and occur after the medication dosage is lowered. And if the medications are used continuously, the brain adapts, and the catamenial pattern may reestablish itself after one or several cycles.

Another AED can be added during the vulnerable period. Benzodiazepines (e.g., lorazepam, clonazepam, clobazam) may be used in this setting. When used for less than 5 days, withdrawal effects (i.e., increased seizure activity after discontinuation) are uncommon but may occur in some patients. Acetazolamide (Diamox), a mild diuretic that inhibits carbonic anhydrase, has been used premenstrually to prevent catamenial exacerbations. Although used for decades, only retrospective and limited evidence supports its use for premenstrual exacerbations (11). Some women with catamenial epilepsy report a benefit from acetazolamide that is reduced over time as tolerance develops. Although some believe that acetazolamide works premenstrually to reduce excess fluid in the brain, acetazolamide has anticonvulsant effects in both men and women for partial and generalized epilepsies (12). Also, while acetazolamide can reduce excess fluid in the brain, it is not clear that this mechanism is related to its efficacy as an AED.

BIRTH CONTROL FOR WOMEN WITH EPILEPSY

Hormonal birth control methods can usually be used safely and effectively for women with epilepsy. There is little evidence for an increase or decrease in seizure frequency when women with epilepsy use hormonal contraception. Oral contraceptive pills can have a higher failure rate when women take certain AED (Table 8.2). The failure rate of the oral contraceptive pill for women with epilepsy taking enzyme-inducing AEDs (e.g., carbamazepine, phenytoin, phenobarbital) is approximately 6% per year. Women with epilepsy who take an enzyme-inducing AED should use an oral contraceptive pill that contains a high dose of estrogen, preferably 50 µg. However, this does not guarantee full contraceptive effect. Similarly, if Depo-Provera is used for birth control in a woman taking an enzyme-inducing AED, more frequent injections (e.g., every 10 weeks instead of every 12 weeks) should be considered. Again, this does not ensure contraceptive efficacy. Recommendations for altering the use of other hormonal birth control methods are not available. The most effective way of preventing pregnancy while

Table 8.2 Antiepileptic Medications and Oral Contraceptives

Should Be Used With Higher-Dose Oral Contraceptives	May Be Used With Any Oral Contraceptives	Level of Antiseizure Medication Is Decreased by Oral Contraceptive
Phenytoin (Dilantin)	Zonisamide (Zonegran)	Lamotrigine (Lamictal)
Primidone (Mysoline)	Valproate (Depakote)	
Carbamazepine (Tegretol, Carbatrol)	Tiagabine (Gabitril)	
Topiramate (Topamax)	Levetiracetam (Keppra)	
Oxcarbazepine (Trileptal)	Ethosuximide (Zarontin)	
Felbamate (Felbatol)		

using hormonal contraception for women with epilepsy is to use it in combination with a barrier method.

Some AEDs have no interactions with birth control pills (e.g., levetiracetam, zonisamide, valproate). Lamotrigine levels decline significantly when taken with oral contraceptives. Therefore, the lamotrigine dose often needs to be increased after a hormonal contraceptive is started and lowered when a contraceptive is discontinued.

SEXUAL FUNCTIONING IN WOMEN WITH EPILEPSY

Most women with epilepsy are satisfied with their sexual lives, but more report reduced interest in sex than women in the general population. Psychological and biological factors may be involved. Women with epilepsy report more anxiety about sexual situations than expected. Some may be anxious that a seizure may occur during sex, while others may fear starting relationships for fear of rejection because of epilepsy-related stigma. However, epilepsy often arises in, or spreads to, limbic and subcortical areas of the brain that modulate sexual desire and response. Sexual dysfunction is more common in women with localization-related (focal) epilepsy than generalized epilepsy (13). The physical sexual response, such as vaginal lubrication, is decreased in women with epilepsy. The cause is unknown.

Some AEDs can cause problems with sexuality. The most problematic are medications with sedative or mood depressant effects, such as phenobarbital and primidone. Sexual side effects can occur with many AEDs (e.g., phenytoin, carbamazepine, valproate, and gabapentin). The cause of sexual side effects may be partly related to the effects of the AEDs, such as phenytoin, on reproductive hormone levels. Hormones like testosterone are important for sexual interest, even in women, as are estradiol and dehydroepiandrosterone (13–14). Finally, depression also increases the risk of problems with sexual function.

The treatment of sexual dysfunction in women with epilepsy has not been well studied. If enzyme-inducing or sedating AEDs are used, medication changes may be worth considering. Drugs traditionally used for male erectile dysfunction, such as sildenafil (Viagra) or tadalafil (Cialis), or testosterone supplementation to enhance performance or libido have not yet been proven effective or safe for women.

INFERTILITY AND EPILEPSY

Women with epilepsy have lower rates of fertility. This likely reflects both a choice by some women because of their epilepsy and their medications. The biological effects of the recurrent seizures, AEDs, and the neurologic disorder that causes epilepsy likely play a role. A biological mechanism is supported by the increased frequency of anovulatory cycles in women with epilepsy when pregnancy is not possible. Other reproductive abnormalities, such as polycystic ovarian syndrome, increased in women with epilepsy and associated with the use of valproate, can also contribute to infertility. No specific AED definitely contributes to or causes infertility. Lower fertility is present only in women (and men) with active epilepsy and not in those who have achieved remission before adulthood (15).

Although current information indicates that women with well-controlled epilepsy have only slightly increased risks for additional problems associated with pregnancy and birth outcomes, some concern still exists on the part of patients and even physicians regarding pregnancy and epilepsy.

PREGNANCY

More than 90% of babies born to women with epilepsy are healthy, although pregnancy poses special issues for these women. Seizure control is critical, and most women must be maintained on an AED during pregnancy. Ideally, women of childbearing age should have their epilepsy reevaluated before conception and get started on folic acid supplementation, although several studies suggest that folate does not reduce the rate of congenital malformations in babies exposed to AEDs during the first trimester (16). Low dose lemotrigine (<300mg/d), and carbamazepine (<400mg/d) are among the safest options in pregnancy. In many cases, it is possible to use only a single AED that has a relatively favorable safety profile for the fetus. However, no AED is proven safe in pregnancy. The rate of major birth defects is 1.6% to 3.2% in the general population and is approximately twice this frequency in babies born to mothers with epilepsy on one AED (4% to 7%) (Table 8.3). The risk of birth defects is increased with AED polytherapy in pregnancy and is highest with the use of valproic acid. A higher dose of one or more drugs also appears to increase the risk of birth defects. All potential changes must be weighed against the risk of increased seizure activity. For example, women who drive face grave risks if they have even one seizure that impairs consciousness. Data for women who conceive on AEP therapy should participate in registries (Table 8.4).

Seizures During Pregnancy

Most women experience no change in seizure frequency or severity during pregnancy, although 20% have an increase in seizure activity, while 20% experience

Table 8.3   Major Malformations in Infants of Women With Epilepsy

Malformation	General Population	Infants of Women With Epilepsy
Congenital heart defect	0.5%	1.5–2%
Cleft lip/palate	0.15%	1.4%
Neural tube defect	0.06%	1–3.8% (VPA) 0.5–1% (CBZ)
Urogenital defect	0.7%	1.7%

Abbreviations: CBZ, carbamazepine; VPA, valproic acid.

Table 8.4   Antiepileptic Drug Pregnancy Registry at Massachusetts General Hospital, Harvard Medical School

If you are pregnant and take antiepileptic drugs (ANTISEIZURE MEDICATIONS), please call TOLL FREE (888)233-2334 to register with the ANTISEIZURE MEDICATIONS Pregnancy Registry. Your identity will remain confidential. More information can be found at http://www.massgeneral.org/antiseizuremedications/

What is the purpose of the Registry?	At present, we lack complete information about the relative safety of specific antiepileptic drugs during pregnancy. The Registry enrolls women over the telephone who are pregnant and taking seizure medications to find answers. As more women register and report the outcome of their pregnancy, the researchers of this registry will be able to identify the safest medications for seizures during pregnancy.
When should I call the Registry?	As early in your pregnancy as possible. It is best to enroll during your 1st trimester, but you can still participate if you are already in your 2nd or 3rd trimester.
How do I register?	By calling toll free (888)233-2334. There are only three telephone interviews: 1. The first call is the longest and can take up to 12 minutes. 2. The registry will call you when you are 7 months pregnant (5 minute call). 3. The registry will call you again after your baby is born (5 minute call).

a decrease in seizures (17–19). Hormonal as well as other physiologic (e.g., sleep deprivation, lower AED levels) and psychological (e.g., stress) changes during pregnancy can alter seizure frequency. Some women reduce or discontinue their AEDs during pregnancy in the mistaken belief that they are simply protecting their child. Although AEDs can cause major and minor congenital malformations, and valproic acid can impair neurodevelopmental outcome, seizures during pregnancy and labor and delivery are not always benign for the fetus or newborn. There must be a balance of the risk of possible seizures and the risk of medications. Generalized tonic-clonic seizures in the mother can lower oxygen levels and raise heart rate in the fetus. Rarely, these seizures, especially status, can cause miscarriage or spontaneous abortion. Even complex partial seizures may cause fetal heart rate changes or distress (20–21). Seizures that cause falls can result in rupture of the membranes protecting the fetus and direct fetal injury.

The management of AEDs during pregnancy often requires frequent monitoring of blood levels. All AED levels decrease during pregnancy, owing to changes in metabolism, protein binding, and body mass. Some medications, such as lamotrigine (Lamictal), are particularly prone to decreased levels in the bloodstream during pregnancy because of changes in how the body metabolizes the drugs. Most of these changes gradually normalize over the first few weeks to months after one's baby is born.

Neurodevelopmental Outcome

Children exposed to AEDs in utero have higher rates of adverse neurodevelopmental outcomes. Children born to women with epilepsy are at increased risk for developmental delay or lower verbal abilities. A variety of factors may contribute to this, including 5 or more convulsive (generalized tonic-clonic) seizures during pregnancy and some AEDs. Intrauterine exposure to valproic acid is associated with the greatest risk of neurodevelopmental problems (22–23), although phenobarbital and phenytoin also appear to be associated with an increased risk of these problems (23). Antiepileptic drug polytherapy for the mother appears to further increase the risk to the fetus. Exposure during the third trimester may be the most detrimental for cognitive outcome.

LABOR, DELIVERY, AND NEWBORN PERIOD

Most women with epilepsy will have a safe vaginal delivery without having a seizure. Having epilepsy and taking AEDs does not limit their options concerning what type of delivery they choose or whether they choose to use pain medication during delivery. The exception to this is meperidine (Demerol); meperidine should be avoided because of its potential to lower the seizure threshold. Only a small fraction of women with epilepsy will have seizures during labor or in the first few days after delivery. However, seizure recurrence may be more likely in women with primary generalized epilepsy, possibly owing to their sensitivity to sleep disruption—and a new baby may mean some sleepless nights.

The newborn period, with its inevitable sleep disruption, can be a time of seizure worsening and may even provoke seizure recurrence for women with previously controlled seizures. Extra precautions should be taken during this time. If their seizures make them likely to drop objects, as occurs with myoclonic seizures or many complex partial seizures, suggest a harness when carrying their babies. If they are likely to fall during a seizure, then using a stroller—even in the house—is an even better option.

Changing time is best done on the floor, rather than on an elevated changing table. Bathing should never be performed alone, as a brief lapse in attention can result in a fatal drowning. The important role that sleep deprivation plays in worsening seizures must be considered. If a woman is breast-feeding, sleep deprivation may be unavoidable. Consider having other adults share the burden of nighttime feedings through the use of formula or harvested breast milk, and the patient should attempt to make up any missed sleep during the baby's daytime naps.

Women with epilepsy on seizure medications do have increased risks for complications, but these risks can be considerably reduced through effective planning prior to pregnancy and careful management during pregnancy and the postpartum period.

Table 8.5   Checklist for Women With Epilepsy Planning or During a Pregnancy

Preconception (prior to pregnancy)	You should be taking the following supplements daily, as suggested by your physician, in addition to your seizure medication(s): 1. Multivitamins or prenatal vitamins 2. Folic acid 0.4–5 mg Discuss with your physician that you are planning a pregnancy and want to transition to the best medication regimen for the safety of you and your developing child. Additional resources: Epilepsy Foundation brochures and Web sites: http://www.efa.org http://www.antiseizuremedicationspregnancyregistry.org/women.htm
Pregnancy	For the duration of your pregnancy, you should be taking the following supplements daily, as prescribed by your physician: 1. Multivitamins or prenatal vitamins 2. Folic acid 0.4–5 mg The level of medication in your blood may decrease during pregnancy. It is recommended that you discuss with your physician regular monitoring of your drug levels during pregnancy and after childbirth. The dose of your seizure medications may be changed based upon the results of your laboratory tests or worsening of seizures, or because of side effects of the medication. It is very important not to miss doses. If you have problems with vomiting within 30 minutes of taking your seizure medication, you should repeat the dose. Your physician will schedule you for a maternal α-fetoprotein and/or "triple screen" at 15–22 weeks gestation. A detailed, structural (level II) ultrasound will be ordered at 16–20 weeks of gestation. This will be performed by a perinatologist. Vitamin K (10 mg daily) may be prescribed beginning at 36 weeks of gestation until delivery to prevent bleeding disorders in the infant, especially for women on phenobarbital. Identify a pediatrician at least 1 month prior to your due date and discuss your plans for breast-feeding. You should discuss a birth plan with your obstetrician and your physician who is prescribing your seizure medication.

(continued)

Table 8.5   Checklist for Women With Epilepsy Planning or During a Pregnancy (*continued*)

Days of Delivery	Take a copy of your birth plan to the hospital. Notify your epilepsy physician of your delivery to help manage any complications or changes in your seizures or in your medication levels.
	Take your seizure medications as directed. Do not miss any in the hospital during labor, delivery, and postpartum.
	Bring an extra supply of your seizure medication with you to the hospital.
	Following delivery, you may be asked to decrease your antiseizure medication.
Please be aware of side effects or other possible complications associated with seizure medications and pregnancy. If you are feeling different from usual, inform your physician.	
If your seizures get worse during your pregnancy, call your physician. If you have a convulsive seizure, contact your obstetrician: you may need to go to the emergency room.	

Abnormalities of baseline endocrine status occur more commonly in people with epilepsy. Abnormalities are most often described for the sex steroid hormone axis, commonly presenting as sexual dysfunction in men and women with epilepsy and lower fertility. Other signs and symptoms in women with epilepsy include menstrual irregularities, premature menopause, and polycystic ovarian syndrome. The evaluation and care of adult people with epilepsy should include considerations of the common hormonal aberrations that occur in this patient population.

Enzyme-inducing AEDs can cause hormonal contraception to fail and can increase the risk of teratogenicity. Higher doses of oral contraceptives can overcome pharmacologic failure but may create additional risks. The effects of reproductive hormones on individual AEDs have recently been clarified, providing helpful guidelines for physicians and patients. Studies show that lamotrigine has a significantly increased clearance (>50%) when used with combined oral contraceptives, which can result in an increased seizure frequency in some patients. Useful alternatives to oral contraceptives include depot injections and intrauterine devices. Subdermal implants are associated with an increased risk of pregnancy in women with epilepsy on enzyme-inducing AEDs. Intrauterine devices and condoms are an alternative to pharmacologic approaches because they lack drug-drug interactions and side effects.

BREAST-FEEDING

Breast-feeding is not associated with known cognitive or neurodevelopmental adverse outcomes (24), although we lack definitive studies. The benefits of breast milk, rich in antibodies and growth factors, must be weighed against the potential negative effects of AEDs that are also present. However, since the child is often exposed to higher levels of AEDs in utero, it is uncertain if the lower concentrations secreted in breast milk, of which only a percentage is absorbed by the newborn's gastrointestinal system, adversely affects the child. Some AED, such as levitiracetam, are excreted at high concentrations in breast milk.

EPILEPSY DURING PERIMENOPAUSE AND MENOPAUSE

Perimenopause, when women produce less estrogen and progesterone and begin to have irregular menses and hot flashes, may be associated with increased seizure activity. In early perimenopause, estrogen levels decline less than progesterone levels, possibly accounting for the reduced seizure threshold. For some women, seizures decrease when they complete menopause (25). These changes in seizure activity during perimenopause and after menopause are more common in women who had catamenial seizures, consistent with hormone-sensitive seizures. Increased seizure activity during perimenopause should be evaluated, and lifestyle factors (e.g. sleep, alcohol use) should be improved, if possible. Increased AED doses may be another consideration.

Women with epilepsy, particularly those with frequent seizures, may experience menopause approximately 4 years earlier than expected (46.5 vs 50.5 years) (26). The cause of this is unknown but may be due to effects of seizures on brain areas that regulate reproductive functioning.

The risks of long-term HRT for postmenopausal women include a small increased risk of breast cancer, dementia, and stroke. This has led to a significant decline in the use of hormone replacement therapy (HRT) (conjugated equine estrogen combined with medroxyprogesterone acetate [Prempro]). However, re-analysis of the data suggests that HRT can lower the risk of dementia and coronary artery disease during the first few years after menopause (27). Therapy with conjugated equine estrogen combined with medroxyprogesterone acetate is associated with a dose-related increase in seizure activity (28). Therefore, HRT should be avoided or monitored carefully in women with epilepsy. If short-term HRT is needed to manage severe hot flashes and other symptoms, estradiol combined with natural progesterone as short-term HRT may be an alternative choice, since natural progesterone may have an antiseizure effect. An adverse effect on seizure frequency with the use of HRT during postmenopause for women with epilepsy was reported in a survey using questionnaires and was later borne out in a clinical trial (29).

FINAL THOUGHTS

Women with epilepsy usually enjoy normal sexual and reproductive function. However, these women face higher rates of decreased libido, infertility, adverse pregnancy outcomes, and other issues such as interactions between contraceptive and AEDs. In most instances, awareness of potential problems and use of strategies to avoid or reduce the impact of these problems can significantly improve health and quality of life.

REFERENCES

1. Herzog AG. Menstrual disorders in women with epilepsy. *Neurology*. 2006;66:S23–28.
2. Smith SS. Estrogen administration increases neuronal responses to excitatory amino acids as a long term effect. *Brain Res*. 1989;503:354–357.
3. Gee KW, McCauley LD, Lan NC. A putative receptor for neurosteroids on the GABA receptor complex: the pharmacological properties and therapeutic potential of epalons. *Crit Rev Neurobiol*. 1995;9:207–227.
4. Reddy DS, Rogawski MA. Neurosteroid replacement therapy for catamenial epilepsy. *Neurotherapeutics*. 2009;6:392–401.
5. Morrell MJ. Epilepsy in women: the science of why it is special. *Neurology*. 1999;53: S42–S48.
6. Herzog AG. Hormonal therapies: progesterone. *Neurotherapeutics*. 2009;6:383–391.
7. Dana Haeri J, Richens A. Effect of norethisterone on seizures associated with menstruation. *Epilepsia*. 1983;24:377–381.
8. Mattson RH, Cramer JA, Caldwell BV, Siconolfi BC. Treatment of seizures with medroxyprogesterone acetate: preliminary report. *Neurology*. 1984;34:1255–1258.
9. Herzog AG. Intermittent progesterone therapy and frequency of complex partial seizures in women with menstrual disorders. *Neurology*. 1986;36:1607–1610.
10. Herzog AG. Progesterone therapy in complex partial and secondary generalized seizures. *Neurology*. 1995;45:1660–1662.
11. Lim LL, Foldvary N, Mascha E, Lee J. Acetazolamide in women with catamenial epilepsy. *Epilepsia*. 2001;42:746–749.
12. Reiss WG, Oles KS. Acetazolamide in the treatment of seizures. *Ann Pharmacother*. 1996;30:514–519.
13. Morrell MJ, Flynn KL, Doñe S, Flaster E, Kalayjian L, Pack AM. Sexual dysfunction, sex steroid hormone abnormalities, and depression in women with epilepsy treated with antiepileptic drugs. *Epilepsy Behav*. 2005;6:360–365.
14. Pack AM. Implications of hormonal and neuroendocrine changes associated with seizures and antiepileptic drugs: a clinical perspective. *Epilepsia*. 2010;51:150–153.
15. Löfgren E, Pouta A, von Wendt L, Tapanainen J, Isojärvi JI, Järvelin MR. Epilepsy in the northern Finland birth cohort 1966 with special reference to fertility. *Epilepsy Behav*. 2009;14:102–107.
16. Morrow JI, Hunt SJ, Russell AJ, et al. Folic acid use and major congenital malformations in offspring of women with epilepsy: a prospective study from the UK Epilepsy and Pregnancy Register. *J Neurol Neurosurg Psychiatry*. 2009;80:506–511.
17. EURAP Study Group. Seizure control and treatment in pregnancy: observations from the EURAP epilepsy pregnancy registry. *Neurology*. 2006;66:354–360.
18. Sabers A. Influences on seizure activity in pregnant women with epilepsy. *Epilepsy Behav*. 2009;15:230–234.
19. Yerby MS, Devinsky O. Epilepsy and pregnancy. *Adv Neurol*. 1994;64:45–63.
20. Nei M, Daly S, Liporace J. A maternal complex partial seizure in labor can affect fetal heart rate. *Neurology*. 1998;51:904–906.
21. Sahoo S, Klein P. Maternal complex partial seizure associated with fetal distress. *Arch Neurol*. 2005;62:1304–1305.

22. Meador K, Reynolds MW, Crean S, Fahrbach K, Probst C. Pregnancy outcomes in women with epilepsy: a systematic review and meta-analysis of published pregnancy registries and cohorts. *Epilepsy Res*. 2008;81:1–13.

23. Bromley RL, Baker GA, Meador KJ. Cognitive abilities and behaviour of children exposed to antiepileptic drugs in utero. *Curr Opin Neurol*. 2009;22:162–166.

24. Meador KJ, Baker GA, Browning N, et al. Effects of breastfeeding in children of women taking antiepileptic drugs. *Neurology*. 2010;75:1954–1960.

25. Harden CL, Pulver MC, Ravdin L, Jacobs AR. The effect of menopause and perimenopause on the course of epilepsy. *Epilepsia*. 1999;40:1402–1407.

26. Harden CL, Koppel BS, Herzog AG, Nikolov BG, Hauser WA. Seizure frequency is associated with age at menopause in women with epilepsy. *Neurology*. 2003;26:451–455.

27. Harden CL. The current state of postmenopausal hormone therapy: update for neurologists and epileptologists. *Epilepsy Curr*. 2007;7:119–122.

28. Harden CL, Herzog AG, Nikolov BG, et al. Hormone replacement therapy in women with epilepsy: a randomized double-blind, placebo-controlled study. *Epilepsia*. 2006;47:1447–1451.

29. Harden CL. Hormone replacement therapy: will it affect seizure control and AED levels? *Seizure*. 2008;17:176–180.

9

Epilepsy: Injury and Prevention

People with epilepsy (PWE) can be injured during seizures or by accidents from associated neurologic impairments, like diminished peripheral vision or poor balance. Therefore, both patients and health care providers should consider the risks of injury as well as work to control seizures. Unfortunately, brief office visits leave little time to explore home or work environments or carefully consider which daily activities, like bathing or exercising, might be made safer. While one can never anticipate all potential dangers, some simple alterations in behavior may prevent injury or, in some cases, be lifesaving. For instance, recommending a low, seated, stationary bike instead of a treadmill to a patient with exercise-induced seizures may prevent a laceration or fracture. Placing nightlights in the bedroom of an elderly patient with unsteady gait from phenytoin-induced neuropathy and ataxia use may prevent falls. Like medication, safety recommendations should be "prescribed" based on seizure type and severity, physical abilities, occupation, age, and other factors.

FALLS

Falls account for most injuries in PWE. Seizures cause falls by diminishing awareness, decreasing leg strength, convulsive movements or impairing coordination and balance. Generalized tonic-clonic seizures frequently cause falls from rapid tonic contraction of muscles and sudden loss of consciousness, but falls may result from complex partial, simple partial, and myoclonic seizures. Atonic seizures, although very brief, cause sudden falls without warning by reducing muscle tone. These dangerous seizures are especially common in people with severe epilepsy and developmental delay.

Seizure-related injuries range from mild contusions, lacerations, and sprains to significant fractures and head traumas. The incidence of injury varies depending on the population studied. Those with severe uncontrolled seizures are at

115

much greater risk than those who are seizure-free. In an Italian study, 5% of patients with recently diagnosed epilepsy had seizure-related accidents over a 1- to 2-year follow-up period (1). Conversely, over a similar period, 62 nursing home patients with multiple disabilities and severe epilepsy fell 2,696 times (2). Six of the falls required serious medical attention.

Fortunately, most seizure-induced falls do not cause serious injury. In a 10-year study of falls in elderly PWE, only 19 injuries resulted from 615 seizures (3). Soft tissue injuries were most frequent, with fractures and intracranial injuries occurring much less often. Seizure-related fractures are usually due to the impact of a fall. However, generalized tonic-clonic seizures may fracture bones from unnatural contortions of the body or from the intense force of muscle contraction on bones and joints. Of 30 fractures in 2,800 patients cared for at one hospital, 15 skull, nasal, and clavicular fractures resulted from seizure-related fall impact; 8 fractures had indeterminate mechanism, and 7 fractures were attributed to the seizures alone. Fractures caused solely by the force of a seizure occurred most frequently in the proximal humerus, with or without an associated shoulder dislocation (4). Vertebral compression fractures may also result from generalized seizures.

Concussions are the most frequent traumatic brain injury from seizure-related falls. Concussions are difficult to diagnose following seizures because postictal states may also cause dizziness, lethargy, headache, nausea, and vomiting. As a result, mild concussions from seizure-related falls may go undiagnosed. One study found that concussion accounted for 10% of accidents seen in those with epilepsy, significantly more than controls (1). More serious brain injuries like epidural, subdural, or intraparenchymal hemorrhages may also result from seizure-related falls (5). Fortunately, the incidence of these life-threatening injuries, even in those with severe epilepsy, is low (2, 6).

BURNS

People with epilepsy experience burns at home at a much higher rate than the general population (7). Most burns are due to seizure-induced falls around stoves, radiators, and in hot showers. Complex partial seizures resulting in diminished awareness may cause patients to burn themselves without falling. An Arizona burn registry cited seizure-related burns in 32 patients over a 5-year period (8). Eleven patients fell onto stoves while cooking; 10 fell on hot pavement; 3 others fell into campfires. Of the burns, 72% were full-thickness burns, and 63% of patients had subtherapeutic antiepileptic medication levels upon admission to the hospital. Seizures while showering may also lead to significant burns. In 3 German patients, seizures causing severe burns while showering were attributed to excessively high water temperatures (9). Shower-related burns could be prevented by using a temperature control that prevents water temperature from rising above a certain level.

Burns due to seizures account for 1.6% to 3.7% of burn unit admissions (10). The only guaranteed strategy to prevent seizure-related falls or burns is to eliminate seizures. Unfortunately, even with the best medical and surgical therapy and a patient who is fully compliant with treatment, seizures can still occur, often unpredictably and in a setting where injury is possible. Although we cannot fully control seizures or injuries that result from seizures, the risk from injury can be reduced. Some recommendations commonly made to reduce falls in the elderly are adaptable for epilepsy. To prevent falls in seniors, the Centers for Disease Control and Prevention recommends home safety improvements, regular exercise, careful medication review, and frequent vision evaluations.

For patients at high risk of falling or of burning themselves, a home safety evaluation of each room may eliminate potential hazards. Table 9.1 provides a list of possible interventions designed to prevent accidents and mitigate the consequence of seizures in the home. Safety assessment and interventions should be tailored for each patient. Recommendations should be based on seizure type, frequency, compliance with treatment, coexisting disabilities, and social factors.

Table 9.1 Home Safety Checklist[a]

General	Install carpet with a heavy pile and underpadding throughout the house, including entrance ways
	Place pads on furniture with sharp corners
	Purchase furniture with rounded corners when possible
	Avoid glass coffee and dining tables
	Close the fireplace screen when there is a fire burning
	PWE with uncontrolled seizures should not be left alone in a room with a fire in a fireplace or the fireplace made safe
	Use electric and home appliance devices that have automatic shutoff switches
	Use chairs that have arms to prevent falls during brief seizures
	Consider a wall-mounted or table top ironing board
	Avoid smoking when alone
	Do not use candles when alone
	Avoid space heaters that tip over
	Make sure motor-driven equipment (e.g., lawn mower) has an automatic shut off

(continued)

Table 9.1   Home Safety Checklist (*continued*)

	Avoid free-standing or table lamps and glass decorations
	Whenever possible, sit down when doing household chores or using tools
	Keep floors clear of clutter and tie up dangling electrical cords
	Avoid climbing up on chairs or ladders
	Put safety gates at the top of steep stairs
	Securely lock outside doors if you tend to wander during a seizure
	If seizures are frequent, consider a helmet or face guard and/or knee or elbow pads, at least when home alone
Bathroom	Doors should open outward (if someone falls against door, it can still be opened)
	Floor should be carpeted with padding underneath
	Avoid locks and use "vacant/occupied" signage
	Take showers rather than baths, if possible
	Place nonskid strips or a rubber bath mat on the floor of the shower
	Ensure that bath or shower drain is always functional prior to use
	Consider shower seat with a safety strap if there is a risk of falling
	Shower when someone else is home
	Keep water levels in the tub low if bathing
	Consider a handheld shower nozzle while seated in tub or shower
	Set water temperature low enough to prevent scalding in the event of loss of consciousness
	Avoid electrical appliances (dryers, razors, curling irons, etc) in the bathroom or near water
	Consider padding edges of tub
	Avoid glass shower doors
	Use shatterproof glass for mirrors
	Consider a padded toilet seat
	Install tub rails or grab bars, if possible

Table 9.1   (*continued*)

	Consider protective covers on faucet handles, nozzles, and the edges of countertops
	Cover radiators or heating units
Kitchen	Use a microwave oven rather than a stove whenever possible
	Cook when someone else is at home
	If using a stove, use back burners only
	Use plastic utensils and containers
	Use cups with lids (commuter or sippy cups) to prevent spills
	Consider using prepared or precut meats to avoid need for knives
	Avoid carrying containers of hot food or liquid (use a cart if possible)
	Wear rubber gloves when washing dishes
	Saucepan handles should face the back of the stove
	Use a stove guard that fits around the side or front of the stove
	Buy a kettle with an automatic shutoff
	Avoid knives, slicers, etc, and use a blender or food processor when possible
Bedroom	Patients with uncontrolled seizures should have roommates, if possible
	Avoid hard-edged bed frames or sharp-cornered bedside tables
	Avoid top bunks
	Avoid potentially suffocating sleeping surfaces (water beds)
	Consider antisuffocation pillows (efficacy still undetermined)
	Consider an audio monitor to alert others to the sounds of a typical seizure
	Seizure alarms triggered by movement or increased heart rate may be helpful to alert others
	Avoid unsecured dental appliances
	Use night lights to prevent falling if wandering postictally

Abbreviation: PWE, people with epilepsy.

[a]The recommendations are for the patients at risk for seizures with loss of consciousness. Not all recommendations will be appropriate for all patients.

Regular exercise reduces fracture risk in the elderly and may help PWE. In a prospective study of elderly women with osteopenia, Finnish researchers showed that exercise reduced postural sway and the rate of falls and fractures (11). Similarly, exercise alone or in combination with vision and/or home hazard reduction was associated with fewer falls in an Australian cohort (12). For those with epilepsy who take antiepileptic drugs (AEDs) that impair balance or cause osteopenia, regular exercise may improve gait stability and strengthen bones, joints, and muscles. This has the potential to reduce the risk of fractures after a fall.

SPORTS-RELATED INJURIES

In a recent Canadian review, PWE were 3 times less likely to experience sports-related injuries than the general population (13). The difference was attributed to a reduction in participation among people with seizure disorders. Despite well-established benefits of exercise for PWE (see Chapter 10), fear of injury sidelines patients. Unfortunately, scant safety data prevent many caregivers from counseling patients confidently about exercise and sports. Detailed studies of epilepsy and injury in sports like hockey, football, basketball, and rugby are lacking. Therefore, physicians must individualize recommendations based on seizure frequency and severity, history of exercise-induced seizures, and level of contact and competition. While concern is warranted for collision sports like football and rugby, no data indicate any additional likelihood of seizures compared with other sports (14).

Concussions are as great a concern for players without as for those with epilepsy. There is an emerging consensus for return to play recommendations for the general population, and this should be applied to those with epilepsy. In general, the player should not return to play the same day of the concussion event. Physical and cognitive assessment is critical before return to play. In children, it is recommended that they be symptom-free for several days before resuming a graduated exercise program (15). However, increasing evidence from boxing- and football-related concussions and repetitive subconcussive head trauma suggests a greater risk of memory impairment later in life (16–17). People with epilepsy who have an increased frequency of memory difficulties may be more sensitive to the long-term effects of minor head traumas. The issue of minor head injuries causing or exacerbating epilepsy has not been well studied. Although epidemiologic studies of minor head injuries suggest that these do not cause epilepsy, anecdotal case series suggest that in some cases, such injuries can cause epilepsy (18–19).

DROWNING AND EPILEPSY

Drowning occurs more frequently in PWE. In a meta-analysis of over 50 studies in the United Kingdom, PWE had a greater than 15-fold chance of drowning risk than the general population (20). The review included swimming and bathing, for the most common sites as submersion injuries are the swimming pool and bathtub. Bathing is especially dangerous in children, where the relative risk of drowning is 96 times higher than that of the general population (21). The risk while swimming is higher in adults, most likely owing to the increased supervision in children. A review of medical examiner investigations of 25 seizure-related drowning deaths over a 10-year period in Alberta, Canada, revealed that 60% occurred in bathtubs (22). Sadly, having a family member at home but not closely supervising did not prevent drowning in several cases. In contrast, only one patient died while taking a shower. Subtherapeutic or undetectable AED levels were found in 23 of the 25 patients, suggesting that seizures were the proximate cause of drowning. Like sudden unexplained death in epilepsy (discussed later in this chapter), postictal respiratory disorders combined with "electrocerebral shutdown," which is associated with impaired arousal and breathing reflexes, contribute to seizure-induced drowning deaths. Two people drowned after falling out of a moving boat. Neither was wearing a personal flotation device.

WATER SAFETY

Drowning is best prevented by meticulous control of seizures and ensuring compliance with AED therapy. For PWE who are still at risk for seizures, especially tonic-clonic seizures, close supervision of bathing and swimming is essential. Children with epilepsy should never bathe alone and should never be left alone in the bathtub, even for brief periods. For older children and adults, showers, preferably with a safety seat and strap, are safest.

People with epilepsy should never swim alone. Murky or open waters should be avoided in favor of supervised pools. Lifeguards should be informed that a swimmer has a seizure disorder. Children and those with uncontrolled seizures should wear life jackets that keep their heads above water when not in a directly supervised swimming class. Bright swimsuits and caps are helpful when observing swimmers with epilepsy.

If a seizure occurs in the water, the patient should first be floated on to his or her back with head and face held out of the water. The patient should then be towed to the shore or the side of the pool and placed on his or her side. The airway should be checked and cleared, and cardiopulmonary resuscitation should be initiated if indicated.

SUDDEN UNEXPLAINED DEATH IN EPILEPSY

Sudden unexplained death in epilepsy (SUDEP) excludes trauma, drowning, status epilepticus, intoxication, or other known causes, but there is often evidence of an associated seizure. SUDEP is often unwitnessed, and the person is often found prone, dead in bed. SUDEP is definite when clinical criteria are met and autopsy reveals no alternative cause of death, such as stroke or myocardial infarction (23).

SUDEP is probable when clinical criteria are met, but there is no autopsy (24). Rates of SUDEP increase with the duration and severity of epilepsy and is much less common in children than adults (25–27). The magnitude of SUDEP is unrecognized by medical or lay communities. In a population-based cohort of children with epilepsy followed for 40 years, SUDEP occurred in 9% of patients and accounted for 38% of all deaths; almost all deaths occurred during adulthood (27). In adults with frequent generalized tonic-clonic seizures (GTCS) poorly controlled epilepsy, the rate of SUDEP can exceed 10% per decade (27–28). The overall population of children with epilepsy has SUDEP rates under 1 per 1,000 patient years, and adults have rates of less than 0.5 to over 9 per 1,000 patient years.

Evidence that terminal seizures are the proximate cause of most SUDEPs is derived from recorded events in epilepsy monitoring units (28–34), case-control studies (27–28), and cases witnessed in the community (28). Other risk factors for SUDEP include early age of epilepsy onset, young adulthood, mental retardation, and major neurologic insult (27–29, 35). Ictal-induced changes in cardiorespiratory function and prolonged suppression of brain activity impairing respiratory drive and arousal responses to hypercapnia and airway obstruction are likely mechanisms leading to death. Epilepsy monitoring unit recordings of SUDEP and near-SUDEP document respiratory problems (i.e., postictal hypoventilation, apnea, cyanosis, inspiratory stridor, laryngospasm, pulmonary edema, and suffocation) cerebral shutdown, and, less often, cardiac arrhythmias (29–33).

PREVENTION OF SUDEP

Although there is no proven way to prevent SUDEP since most SUDEP events occur after seizures, seizure control is considered the first line of SUDEP prevention. Ensuring compliance with AEDs with therapeutic blood monitoring and medication reminders is valuable in patients with break-through seizures. Other strategies to enhance compliance are the use of weekly pill boxes; extra supplies of medication distributed in places where a patient may be or will have ready access (e.g., work, backpack, purse); creating a routine for taking AEDs (e.g., after brushing one's teeth in the morning, before getting into bed at night); plans for making up for missed medication; and so on. For patients with continued seizures despite numerous AED trials, alternative treatments must be considered. Epilepsy surgery for medically refractory seizures originating in resectable regions of cortex may fully control seizures and can reduce the risk of SUDEP when seizures are well controlled (36–38).

Unfortunately, aside from controlling seizures either medically or surgically, strategies for SUDEP prevention are relatively theoretical. Analysis of the circumstances of SUDEP cases indicates that some simple measures may be helpful. Most SUDEP occurs when patients are alone. Additionally, nearly half of patients are found in bed, and most are found in the prone position

(39). If possible, patients at high risk for SUDEP (e.g., those with tonic-clonic seizures or nocturnal seizures) should have a roommate or supervision (40). Supervision can include a listening device to detect the sounds of a convulsive seizure or seizure alarms that detect motion in the bed. Currently available seizure alarms have not been rigorously studied but are modest in cost (e.g. $150 for SmartWatch and $300 for the MedPage MP5 Bed Movement Epilepsy Seizure Alarm, available on Amazon.com). Antisuffocation pillows that allow for continued respirations even when a patient is lying prone http:// esuk.uk.com/index.php?option=com_content&view=article&id=6&Itemid= 170 are sensible but remain unproven in SUDEP prevention.

DRIVING AND EPILEPSY

Seizures while driving are an important public safety concern. State laws deny the privilege to drive in those individuals who have experienced seizures that impair consciousness or motor control during the prior 3 to 12 months. The precise criteria for restricting driving vary by state and include not only the duration of being seizure-free, but also, in some states, whether the individual has a reliable aura before the seizure progresses, or if the seizures occur only in sleep or shortly after awakening, etc. Unfortunately, many individuals with poorly controlled seizures drive. In a multicenter epilepsy surgery study, over 30% of 367 patients had driven in the last year (41). Younger individuals and men were more likely to drive. At some time in the past, 144 of the 367 individuals had one or more seizures while driving: 98 experienced at least one seizure-related accident; 94% reported property damage; 32% had an injury; and 20% caused injury to others (41). Seizure-related motor vehicle accidents (MVAs) are likely to be underreported (42). Mandatory seizure-free periods required by state governments vary, as does the physician's role in counseling and supervising a patient's driving (43). Many patients do not receive proper counseling and accurate information from their physicians about driving with epilepsy (44).

PREVENTING SEIZURE-RELATED MOTOR VEHICLE ACCIDENTS

Prevention of seizure-related MVAs is based largely on risk assessment and proper counseling. Seizure-related MVAs are less likely to occur after 1 year of seizure freedom, in patients with the same aura before all seizures, in those without prior MVAs, and in the absence of recent medication changes or missed doses (43).

While no duration of seizure freedom guarantees safety from seizure-related MVAs, appropriate counseling about state laws and restrictions on driving may help keep high-risk drivers off the road. Documenting AED levels and compliance in patients with prior accidents even after a specified seizure-free period has passed may also be helpful. Finally, urging all patients with past seizures to avoid driving when overtired, sleep deprived, under excessive stress, or ill may be lifesaving.

OTHER DANGERS

A recent Canadian study compared a large group of PWE with others in the general population. After controlling for medical and psychiatric comorbidities, PWE did not have higher suicide or motor vehicle rates, but were more likely to be assaulted than those in the general population (45). Notably, before adjustment for comorbid disorders, the group with epilepsy had a relative risk of 1.83 for MVAs and 4.32 for attempted or completed suicide. These risks declined after factoring in comorbid disorders, and although the risks were higher than in the general population (1.32 to 1.38), they did not reach statistical significance. This study highlights the risk of PWE for assault or robbery, likely when their level of consciousness or responsiveness is impaired during or after a seizure. To reduce this risk, individuals with seizures that impair consciousness or motor control should avoid traveling alone in neighborhoods with high crime rates, avoid wearing jewelry (especially expensive types), conceal items like iPods, and so on. Common sense and forethought are essential.

REFERENCES

1. Beghi E, Cornaggia C, RESt-1 Group. Morbidity and accidents in patients with epilepsy: results of a European cohort study. *Epilepsia*. 2002;43:1076–1083.
2. Nakken KO, Lossius R. Seizure-related injuries in multihandicapped patients with therapy-resistant epilepsy. *Epilepsia*. 1993;34:836–840.
3. Lees A. Retrospective study of seizure-related injuries in older people: a 10-year observation. *Epilepsy Behav*. 2010;19:441–444.
4. Finelli PF, Cardi JK. Seizure as a cause of fracture. *Neurology*. 1989;39:858–860.
5. Zwimpfer TJ, Brown J, Sullivan I, Moulton RJ. Head injuries due to falls caused by seizures: a group at high risk for traumatic intracranial hematomas. *J Neurosurg*. 1997; 86:433–437.
6. Russell-Jones DL, Shorvon SD. The frequency and consequences of head injury in epileptic seizures. *J Neurol Neurosurg Psychiatry*. 1989;52:659–662.
7. Ansari Z, Brown K, Carson N. Association of epilepsy and burns—a case control study. *Aust Fam Physician*. 2008;37:584–589.
8. Rimmer RB, Bay RC, Foster KN, et al. Thermal injury in patients with seizure disorders: an opportunity for prevention. *J Burn Care Res*. 2007;28:318–323.
9. Unglaub F, Woodruff S, Demir E, Pallua N. Patients with epilepsy: a high-risk population prone to severe burns as a consequence of seizures while showering. *J Burn Care Rehabil*. 2005;26:526–528.
10. Wirrell EC. Epilepsy-related injuries. *Epilepsia*. 2006;47:79–86.
11. Korpelainen R, Keinänen-Kiukaanniemi S, Nieminen P, Heikkinen J, Väänänen K, Korpelainen J. Long-term outcomes of exercise: follow-up of a randomized trial in older women with osteopenia. *Arch Intern Med*. 2010;170:1548–1556.
12. Fitzharris MP, Day L, Lord SR, Gordon I, Fildes B. The Whitehorse No Falls trial: effects on fall rates and injurious fall rates. *Age Ageing*. 2010;39:728–733.
13. Téllez-Zenteno JF, Hunter G, Wiebe S. Injuries in people with self-reported epilepsy: a population-based study. *Epilepsia*. 2008;49:954–961.

14. Sahoo SK, Fountain NB. Epilepsy in football players and other land-based contact or collision sport athletes: when can they participate, and is there an increased risk? *Curr Sports Med Rep*. 2004;3:284–288.

15. Purcell L. What are the most appropriate return-to-play guidelines for concussed child athletes? *Br J Sports Med*. 2009;43:i51–i55.

16. Ravdin LD, Barr WB, Jordan B, Lathan WE, Relkin NR. Assessment of cognitive recovery following sports related head trauma in boxers. *Clin J Sport Med*. 2003;13:21–27.

17. Guskiewicz KM, Marshall SW, Bailes J, et al. Association between recurrent concussion and late-life cognitive impairment in retired professional football players. *Neurosurgery*. 2005;57:719–726.

18. Annegers JF, Grabow JD, Groover RV, et al. Seizures after head trauma: a population study. *Neurology*. 1980;30:683–689.

19. Devinsky O. Epilepsy after minor head trauma. *J Epilepsy*. 1996;9:94–97.

20. Bell GS, Gaitatzis A, Bell CL, Jonson AL, Sander JW. Drowning in people with epilepsy: how great is the risk? *Neurology*. 2008;71:578–582.

21. Diekema DS, Quan L, Holt VL. Epilepsy as a risk factor for submersion injury in children. *Pediatrics*. 1993;91:612–616.

22. Ryan CA, Dowling G. Drowning deaths in people with epilepsy. *CMAJ*. 1993;148:781–784.

23. Nashef L. Sudden unexpected death in epilepsy: terminology and definitions. *Epilepsia*. 1997;38:S6–S8.

24. Annegers JF. United States perspective on definitions and classifications. *Epilepsia*. 1997;38:S9–S12.

25. Camfield CS, Camfield PR, Veugelers PJ. Death in children with epilepsy: a population-based study. *Lancet*. 2002;359:1891–1895.

26. Donner EJ, Smith CR, Snead OC III. Sudden unexplained death in children with epilepsy. *Neurology*. 2001;57:430–434.

27. Sillanpaa M, Shinnar S. Long-term mortality in childhood-onset epilepsy. *N Engl J Med*. 2010;363:2522–2529.

28. Tomson T, Nashef L, Ryvlin P. Sudden unexpected death in epilepsy: current knowledge and future directions. *Lancet Neurol*. 2008;7:1021–1031.

29. Tao JX, Qian S, Baldwin M, et al. SUDEP, suspected positional airway obstruction, and hypoventilation in postictal coma. *Epilepsia*. 2010;51:2344–2347.

30. Thomas P, Landre E, Suisse G, Breloin J, Dolisi C. Syncope anoxo-ischemique par dyspnae obstructive au cours d'une crise partielle complexe temporale droite. *Epilepsies*. 1996;54:258–258.

31. Bateman LM, Spitz M, Seyal M. Ictal hypoventilation contributes to cardiac arrhythmia and SUDEP: report on two deaths in video-EEG–monitored patients. *Epilepsia*. 2010;51:916–920.

32. Bird JM, Dembny KAT, Sandeman D, Butler S. Sudden unexplained death in epilepsy: an intracranially monitored case. *Epilepsia*. 1997;38:S52–S56.

33. Espinosa PS, Lee JW, Tedrow UB, Bromfield EB, Dworetzky BA. Sudden unexpected near death in epilepsy: malignant arrhythmia from a partial seizure. *Neurology*. 2009;72(19):1702–1703.

34. So E, Sam M, Lagerlund T. Postictal central apnea as a cause of SUDEP: evidence from a near-SUDEP incident. *Epilepsia*. 2000;41:1494–1497.

35. Asadi-Pooya AA, Sperling MR. Clinical features of sudden unexpected death in epilepsy. *J Clin Neurophysiol*. 2009;26:297–301.

36. Hennessy MJ, Langan Y, Elwes RD, Binnie CD, Polkey CE, Nashef L. A study of mortality after temporal lobe epilepsy surgery. *Neurology*. 1999;53:1276–1283.

37. Nilsson L, Ahlbom A, Farahmand BY, Tomson T. Mortality in a population-based cohort of epilepsy surgery patients. *Epilepsia*. 2003;44:575–581.
38. Sperling MR, Harris A, Nei M, Liporace JD, O'Connor MJ. Mortality after epilepsy surgery. *Epilepsia*. 2005;46:49–53.
39. Kloster R, Engelskjøn T. Sudden unexpected death in epilepsy (SUDEP): a clinical perspective and a search for risk factors. *Neurol Neurosurg Psychiatry*. 1999;67:439–444.
40. Langan Y, Nashef L, Sander JW. Case-control study of SUDEP. *Neurology*. 2005;64: 1131–1133.
41. Berg AT, Vickrey BG, Sperling MR, et al. Driving in adults with refractory localization-related epilepsy. Multi-Center Study of Epilepsy Surgery. *Neurology*. 2000;54:625–630.
42. Friedman DE, Gilliam FG. Seizure-related injuries are underreported in pharmacoresistant localization-related epilepsy. *Epilepsia*. 2010;51:43–47.
43. Krauss GL, Krumholz A, Carter RC, Li G, Kaplan P. Risk factors for seizure-related motor vehicle crashes in patients with epilepsy. *Neurology*. 1999;52:1324–1329.
44. Drazkowski JF, Neiman ES, Sirven JI, McAbee GN, Noe KH. Frequency of physician counseling and attitudes toward driving motor vehicles in people with epilepsy: comparing a mandatory-reporting with a voluntary-reporting state. *Epilepsy Behav*. 2010;19:52–54.
45. Kwon C, Liu M, Quan H, Thoo V, Wiebe S, Jetté N. Motor vehicle accidents, suicides, and assaults in epilepsy: a population-based study. *Neurology*. 2011;76:801–806.

10

Enhancing Cognition

Memory and other cognitive problems are common in epilepsy, often resulting from underlying brain disorders, seizures, and antiepileptic medications. Many disorders that cause epilepsy—such as head injury, stroke, infection, and tumor—injure the brain and cause enduring structural lesions. Cognitive recovery after brain injury often extends over months and years, but seizures can interrupt recovery, causing plateaus and regressions. The negative effects of epilepsy on cognitive function have been challenging to untangle from other factors, such as medication, underlying brain disorder, and comorbid cognitive disorders such as attention deficit disorder (ADD). Seizures often contribute to a multifactorial problem.

The epileptogenic disorder of function is a model of epilepsy as a continuous disorder of brain function (1). We view seizures as the only symptom of epilepsy, but that is an illusion. Seizures are brief periods of maximal neuronal dysfunction that are associated with more persistent and even nonparoxysmal disorders of function. A dramatic example is Landau-Kleffner syndrome, where seizures are typically rare and easily controlled, but the nearly continuous epilepsy wave activity in sleep severely impairs language and other cognitive functions.

Recurrent seizures should not be underestimated. Seizure burden—the cumulative measure of seizure severity, seizure frequency, and duration of epilepsy—may correlate with long-term cognitive and behavioral consequences. Although patients are often told that seizures do not injure the brain, recurrent tonic-clonic seizures can cause irreversible structural and function damage. Big seizures, long seizures, recurrent seizures, and relentless continuity of interictal epilepsy waves can sum, perhaps exponentially, to disrupt function and injure structure. Individual susceptibility likely accounts for the wide variance in how seizures and epilepsy affect different people, yet over time, negative effects often accumulate.

Despite the best rehabilitative and medical care, cognitive problems plague many people with epilepsy. Deficits can involve attention, memory, executive functions (working memory, planning, judgment, reasoning), mathematical skill, visuospatial functions, and other mental functions. Some faculties, such as attention and language, form cognitive foundations. If you do not pay attention, then you do not understand, learn, or remember. A selective impairment of attention can falsely suggest global dysfunction. Similarly, impaired language comprehension can lead to errors on verbal tests and even visuospatial tests given with verbal instructions. One of the most critical cognitive functions—social function—is often difficult to quantify and so often eludes identification by neuropsychological or neurologic evaluation, yet it may be the most disabling problem.

DEFINE THE PROBLEM

The severity and scope of cognitive impairment should be defined. Neuropsychological evaluation assesses a broad range of cognitive and behavioral functions and compares performance with age-matched normative data. Defining strengths and weaknesses allows identification of cognitive domains to target in therapy, and strengths can be tapped to assist weaker functions. The testing provides a baseline to assess the beneficial impact of therapy as well as the negative effects of medication, seizures, aging, and other insults. Since cognitive and behavioral problems often coexist and interface, psychiatric and psychological assessment is often helpful.

EXAMINE THE CURRENT THERAPY

In evaluating people with epilepsy with cognitive problems, the first consideration should be subtracting a toxic drug rather than adding a supplement or drug. Drugs such as phenobarbital, topiramate, phenytoin, and others can impair cognitive function. Problems are often dose related, so dose reductions can be helpful. Ideally, one should eliminate a cognitively toxic drug if possible. "Cognitively benign drugs" such as lamotrigine can cause cognitive impairment in very sensitive individuals at standard doses, and with very high doses, the drugs often impair cognition. Even when the antiepileptic drug (AED) regimen minimizes adverse effects and maximizes therapeutic effects, cognition may be impaired. What is the role for other nonpharmacologic strategies, supplements, or medications in improving cognitive function?

CONSIDER NONPHARMACOLOGIC APPROACHES

Traditionally, cognitive problems were treated with speech and cognitive therapies, while physical problems were treated with physical (gross motor) and occupational (fine motor) therapy. Although these safe, intuitively helpful therapies are the standard of care and uniformly endorsed by almost all patients and families, the efficacy of speech and cognitive therapies are not well established in controlled trials. Many studies are underpowered (2). For example, after stroke, patients with aphasia who receive speech therapy have similar outcomes as those who interact with trained volunteers (3). Similarly, intensive speech therapy was not more effective than regular speech therapy after stroke (4). Thus, spontaneous recovery (healing, use of alternate structures and pathways) after stroke may be critical. Human contact that exercises the impaired faculty in a supportive and progressive manner may be more important than the "specific technique."

Randomized controlled trials (RCTs) support specific recommendations to improve language and perception after stroke and to improve attention, memory, functional communication, and executive functioning after head injury (5). These strategies include the following: (a) strengthen or relearn behavioral patterns learned before the injury; (b) develop novel, compensatory cognitive approaches that tap preserved functions; (c) use external mechanisms to help compensate for weakness (e.g., hand electronic devices to make notes and remind one of appointments and medication schedules, environmental structuring); and (d) even where deficits cannot be compensated, help people understand the problems and psychologically adapt to them (5). Cognitive impairment in epilepsy, head injury, Alzheimer disease, and many other neurologic disorders may be accompanied by depression. Psychological and pharmacologic therapy for depression can improve not only mood but also quality of life and cognition.

Computerized programs can stimulate mental activity and potentially help prevent or reverse memory and other cognitive disorders. The Advanced Cognitive Training for Independent and Vital Elderly trial found that cognitive training improved basic mental abilities, health-related quality of life, and performance of activities of daily life 5 years after training. Unfortunately, patients with mild cognitive impairment did not benefit from memory training but improved in their reasoning and processing speed (6). Sadly, those who need it most may benefit least.

DRUGS AND SUPPLEMENTS TO ENHANCE COGNITIVE FUNCTION

Ingestion of substances to enhance cognitive function presents more questions than answers. What drugs and supplements improve cognitive function? How strong is the evidence of efficacy? What percentage of healthy versus patient populations benefit? How much is the benefit? How sustained is the benefit? Is a statistically significant effect a clinically significant effect? What are the potential side effects? If supplements or drugs improve cognition, should everyone take them? All of us would like to enhance attention, working memory, creativity, writing skills, mental processing speed, and social skills. Patient populations may be more vulnerable to side effects. Although supplements are reported to be natural and healthy, many can alter liver metabolism and the effects of other central nervous system drugs. In other cases, supplements may alter the natural balance within the body. For example, amino acids compete with one another for absorption into the brain. If large amounts of one or two amino acids are consumed in supplements, absorption of other amino acids may be reduced.

Nootropics (smart drugs, cognitive enhancers) are composed of a range of substances that are believed to benefit memory, cognition, attention, and other mental capacities. These substances include drugs, supplements, functional foods, and nutraceuticals. Originally, nootropics were defined by the following criteria: (a) enhance learning and memory; (b) prevent loss of learned information and behaviors after exposure to disruptive stressors (e.g., hypoxia, electrically induced convulsions); (c) protect the brain from physical trauma or chemical (e.g., sco-polamine) toxins; (d) increase the efficiency of tonic control mechanisms in the cortex and subcortex; and (e) have little or no toxicity or side effects (e.g., motor hyperactivity, agitation, anxiety, sedation) commonly seen with other psycho-active drugs (7). While nootropics are "substances that improve cognitive func-tion," cognitive enhancers (e.g., methylphenidate, memantine) are not necessarily nootropics. The proposed mechanisms of nootropic action include the following: (a) supplying vital nutrients that the brain uses to synthesize neurotransmitters, hormones, enzymes, and other compounds; (b) increase the supply of oxygen to the brain; (c) stimulate neural growth processes; or (d) protect the brain against stress or injury.

Data supporting the efficacy of cognitive enhancers are limited, with the greatest evidence for drugs approved by the U.S. Food and Drug Administration (FDA) for ADD, narcolepsy, and dementia. Double-blind RCTs establish the efficacy of these drugs, yet these data generate controversy in lay and profes-sional communities. Should we medicate behavior in children? How well did those studies assess difficult-to-measure side effects such as "flattening of per-sonality" or "feeling different than yourself" on stimulants? Since most RCTs are short term, how well have we established the safety of long-term use of these drugs, especially in children? Since many of the RCTs were well powered, does a statistically significant finding translate into a clinically significant benefit? These issues are relevant to FDA-approved as well as other therapies.

TREATING ATTENTION DISORDERS

Stimulants were introduced in the 1930s (amphetamine) to treat nasal conges-tion and obesity. Amphetamines were used extensively in World War II by the Germans and British to increase attention and combat fatigue. After the war, the addictive potential and behavioral toxicity associated with high doses were rec-ognized, and access to these medications was limited. They were subsequently found to be very effective in treating a range of symptoms in ADD and attention deficit/hyperactivity disorder (ADHD).

Attention deficit/hyperactivity disorder is treated with 2 categories of medications: stimulants and amoxetine non-stimulants. Stimulants comprise methylphenidates (Ritalin, Concerta, Vyvanse, Metadate) and amphetamines (Dexadrine, Adderall); nonstimulants include amoxetine (Strattera) and guan-facine (Intuniv). Nonmedical changes such as having the child sit in the first row in school can be quite helpful. Cognitive and behavioral therapies can be beneficial and often provide additional benefits to medication (8–9). There is no evidence that chiropractic treatment improves ADHD (10). When the educational and social problems significantly impair quality of life, medications should be considered. Stimulants paradoxically relax children and help them focus their minds. Stimulants can be used safely in children for prolonged periods but must be carefully supervised by a physician. Side effects include decreased appetite and weight loss, stomach discomfort, difficulty sleeping, depression, personality changes (e.g., quieter, social withdrawal), and mood changes (e.g., anxiety, irritability). Although the dose of stimulants must often be increased as the child ages to compensate for body and liver growth, in many cases, a gradual reduction is possible, as the disorder lessens with age.

Other drugs may improve ADHD symptoms. These include atomoxetine, guanfacine, modafinil, selegiline, and nicotine patch (11–15). Clonidine has only case series to support its use, and bupropion should be avoided. Atomoxetine and guanfacine are nonstimulant alternatives to treat ADD and ADHD. They can be safely used in people with epilepsy. They have fewer side effects (does not suppress appetite or growth and does not cause insomnia), but many find it less effective than stimulants. A review of clinical trial and postmarketing experience with atomoxetine did not show evidence of an increased seizure risk (16). Atomoxetine is also effective for patients with ADHD with comorbid disorders such as oppositional defiant disorder (12).

Epilepsy and ADHD are bidirectionally related (17). In children with epilepsy, ADHD is a common comorbid disorder. Among children with new-onset idiopathic epilepsy, 31% had ADHD versus 6% of controls, and usually antedated epilepsy (18). Other studies also found increased rates of ADHD among people with epilepsy at diagnosis (21%) and after 1 year (42%) (19). The presence of ADHD after 1 year was associated with active seizures for at least 6 months, persisting interictal epileptiform abnormalities, and emotional and behavioral disorders at diagnosis (19). Conversely, children with ADHD have a 2.5 to 2.7 times greater chance of developing epilepsy than those without ADHD (20–21). Proposed mechanisms for the bidirectional relation between epilepsy and ADHD include attention side effects of AEDs (phenobarbital, gabapentin, vigabatrin, and topiramate); shared effects of the underlying neurodevelopmental disorder; effects of chronic seizures and subclinical epileptiform activity, adrenergic dysfunction, and common genetic disorders; and genetics.

Children with epilepsy and comorbid ADHD have higher rates of academic underachievement and impairments in neuropsychological and parental measures of executive function (18). Quantitative magnetic resonance imaging in children with ADHD reveals increased gray matter in the frontal lobe and decreased brainstem volume (18). Symptoms of ADHD are more common in frontal lobe epilepsy, childhood absence epilepsy, and benign rolandic epilepsy. In many cases, the symptoms antedate seizure onset (22).

Stimulants are effective in treating ADHD symptoms in people with epilepsy (17, 23). There is much lore but little information about the safety of methylphenidate in people with epilepsy. We lack controlled and well-powered trials to detect changes in seizure frequency associated with methylphenidate use. The *Physicians' Desk Reference*, the standard guide to medical drugs that houses all of the "package inserts" approved by drug companies and the FDA, discourages the use of methylphenydate in people with epilepsy or epileptiform abnormalities on electroencephalogram (24). Stimulants can be used safely in most children and adults with epilepsy. Insomnia, a potential side effect of stimulants, may increase seizure activity. Methylphenidate is well tolerated by most people with epilepsy (25–28). There was no increase in seizure activity in patients with well-controlled epilepsy, but there may be in those with active seizures (23, 29).

The safety of methylphenidate and other stimulants must be weighed against the impact of ADHD on the child or adult with epilepsy. There are extremely little data regarding the danger or safety of amphetamine use in epilepsy. Notably, the *Physicians' Desk Reference* does not list epilepsy as a relative or absolute contraindication to the use of dextroamphetamine and amphetamine (Dexedrine, Adderall). In an insurance company database with more than 30,000 patients with ADHD, use of stimulants and atomoxetine were not associated with an increased risk of seizures (30). We simply lack data, but the general clinical consensus is that these drugs are safe in children with epilepsy.

Guanfacine (Tenex and Intuniv) is an α_{2A} receptor agonist, FDA-approved for ADD and ADHD. The recently available extended-release preparation better tolerated and more effective in reducing inattention, hyperactivity, impulsivity, and oppositional behavior (31). The most common side effect of guanfacine is tiredness, but this is reduced by the extended-release formulations and improves with time. In pilot studies of patients with localization-related epilepsy, guanfacine improved attentional memory tasks, with slightly greater benefits in patients with frontal than in those with temporal lobe epilepsy (32). Guanfacine does not appear to increase the risk of seizures. Impulsivity is a common feature of ADHD, and it can independently affect a child's social relations and academic achievements. The tendency to automatically react to environmental stimuli leads to problems, since reflection is bypassed and consequences are not considered. The ability to reflect on one's actions and consider both short-term and long-term effects is only fully achieved in adulthood. Stimulants, atomoxetine (Strattera), guanfacine (Tenex; Intuniv), and clonidine (Catapress) can reduce impulsivity. Clonidine and guanfacine can cause sedation but do not lessen seizure control.

TREATING MEMORY DISORDERS

The most common disorder associated with serious memory and other cognitive problems is Alzheimer disease. It is also the only disorder for which large RCTs demonstrate the efficacy of medication to enhance cognitive function and slow disease progression. Unfortunately, in people with epilepsy, we lack RCTs of the medications (cholinesterase [ChE] inhibitors [ChEIs] and neuromuscular blocking agent receptor antagonists) that improve cognition in Alzheimer disease. Since Alzheimer disease involves the relatively selective loss of cholinergic neurons, there is less theoretical basis for the ChEIs in other diseases. Since acetylcholine (ACh) is involved in learning and memory, enhancing cholinergic activity in the brain could theoretically improve these functions in neurologically impaired and healthy individuals. We have limited data, but an NMDA receptor antagonist like memantine does not improve cognitive performance in patients with multiple sclerosis (33).

CHOLINESTERASE INHIBITORS (ChEIs)

In Alzheimer disease, there is a progressive loss of basal forebrain neurons that synthesize ACh, causing a cortical and subcortical deficiency of ACh. Since the postsynaptic cholinergic cells and their receptors are relatively spared, ChEIs increase intrasynaptic ACh, which enhances postsynaptic stimulation. The efficacy of ChEIs is limited by progressive loss of cholinergic neurons and postsynaptic cells and generalized cell loss.

The only cognitive enhancers approved to treat Alzheimer disease are the 4 ChEIs and memantine (Table 10.1). In RCTs, ChEIs modestly improve quality of life, activities of daily living, and behavioral/neuropsychological/global outcomes. No trials directly compare ChEIs, but data suggest similar modest efficacy for the different drugs. The main side effects of ChEIs are nausea, cramping, diarrhea, and vomiting. Since tacrine has hepatic toxicity, it is rarely used. Several ChEIs enhance REM sleep, which may contribute to their efficacy.

Tacrine

Tacrine inhibits ACh binding to ChE, increases cholinergic activity at muscarinic and nicotinic receptors, and increases ACh release. It is extensively metabolized by the p450 system in the liver. Liver function tests should be obtained every other week while the dose is increased and then every 3 months thereafter. Hepatic toxicity is dose-dependent and usually reversible. Randomized controlled trials with doses up to 160 mg/d for 2 to 12 months showed cognitive skill improvements in 15% to 30% of patients with senile dementia of the Alzheimer type (SDAT) (34–35). Tacrine does not appear to benefit patients with non-SDAT dementias or advanced SDAT.

Donepezil

Donepezil reversibly and noncompetitively inhibits ChE and dose-dependently increases brain extracellular ACh. Common side effects are gastrointestinal (GI) and, less often, muscle cramps, insomnia, fatigue, and anorexia. An initial dose of 5 mg at bedtime can be effective. Ten milligrams once daily produces clinically insignificant cognitive improvements over 5 mg/day, but GI toxicity is more common. An initial trial of 5 mg daily should be undertaken before increasing to

Table 10.1 Pharmacologic Properties of Cognitive Enhancers

Compound (Class)	Enzyme Selectivity	Effect of Food on Absorption	Delay to Peak Serum Level (h)	Half-Life (h)	Protein Binding (%)	Hepatic Metabolism	Availability	Dosing
Anticholinesterase								
Tacrine (acrinidine)	ButyrylChE > AcetylChE	Delays	1–2.5	2–4	75	CYP1A2 CYP2D6	10-, 20-, 30-, and 40-mg tablets	Start 10 mg qid. Titrate by 10 mg qid x 4 wk to 40 mg qid.
Donepezil (piperidine)	AcetylChE	None	3–5	70	95	CYP2D6 CYP3A4	5- and 10-mg tablets	Start 5 mg HS. Titrate to 10 mg HS.
Rivastigmine (carbamate)	AcetylChE = ButyrylChE	Delays	0.5–1.5	10	40	None	1.5-, 3-, 4-, 5-, and 6-mg tablets; 2 mg/mL syp	Start 1.5 mg bid. Increase by 1.5 mg per dose q 2 wk up to 6-12 mg bid.
Galantamine (phenanthrene alkaloid)	AcetylChE; modulates nicotininc	Delays	0.5–1.0	5–6	15	CYP2D6 CYP3A4	4-, 8-, and 12-mg tablets	Start 4 mg bid. Escalate dose q 4 wk up to 16-32 mg/d.
MAO-B Inhibitor								
Selegiline	MAO-B >> MAO-A	Increased bioavailability	0.5–1.5	10			5-mg tablets	5 mg qam and q noon.
Cyclic GABA inhibitor								
Piracetam (acetamide)	None		0.5–1.0	5–6		None	800-mg tablets (not available in United States)	Start 2–4 grams tid. Increase to a maximum of 18–24 g/d over 2 wk.

Abbreviations: bid, twice a day; ChE - cholintesterase; GABA, γ-aminobutyric acid; HS, every night; MAO, monoamine oxidase; q, each; qam, every morning; qid, 4 times a day; SYP - syrup.

10 mg daily. Donepezil is effective for early-onset as well as advanced SDAT for up to 2 years. In people with epilepsy and traumatic brain injury–related cognitive impairment, preliminary data suggest that donepezil leads to mild memory improvements but does not increase seizure risk (36–37). Depression predicts the progression from amnestic mild cognitive impairment to Alzheimer disease (38). Treatment with donepezil delays the cognitive deterioration in depressed patients with amnestic mild cognitive impairment (38).

Rivastigmine

Rivastigmine is a noncompetitive ChEI that preferentially inhibits ChE form G1, which is found in high levels in Alzheimer brains. Rivastigmine treatment has efficacy in mild to moderate Alzheimer disease. In addition to GI effects, other adverse effects include dizziness, fatigue, agitation, loss of appetite, asthenia, and diaphoresis. It should be cautiously used in cardiovascular/pulmonary disease, diabetes mellitus, GI diseases, urogenital tract obstruction, and Parkinson disease (may exacerbate motor symptoms.) Dose adjustments are not required in hepatically and renally impaired patients. It is primarily metabolized by ChEs; it does not induce the p450 system and has few drug interactions.

Galantamine

Galantamine is a reversible, competitive ChEI that also amplifies ACh effects at presynaptic and postsynaptic nicotinic receptors. Galantamine can improve mild to moderate dementia with doses of 16 to 24 mg/d, showing sustained effects on cognition, activities of daily life, sleep quality, and behavior.

N-METHYL D-ASPARTIC ACID RECEPTOR ANTAGONISTS: MEMANTINE

Memantine blocks the *N*-methyl D-aspartic acid glutamate receptor and is approved to treat moderate to severe Alzheimer disease. Notably, the United Kingdom's National Institute for Clinical Experience does not recommend memantine since it has limited benefits and a high cost (39). Memantine provides a small but beneficial effect on cognition, mood, behavior, and the ability to perform daily activities in moderate to severe Alzheimer disease (40). Side effects are infrequent but include dizziness, drowsiness, headache, insomnia, confusion, agitation, and hallucinations. Rarely, vomiting, cystitis, and increased libido can occur.

In Alzheimer disease, the combination of ChEIs and memantine is superior to ChEIs or placebo alone in regard to cognitive improvement and delay of admission to the nursing home (41–42).

DRUGS AND SUPPLEMENTS THAT ARE NOT APPROVED BY THE FDA

Piracetam

Piracetam is a cyclic γ-aminobutyric acid derivative that can reduce myoclonus and may have cognitive enhancing and neuroprotective properties (43). It is not available in the United States but can be legally imported, and its use is not regulated. Its mechanism of action is unknown but may involve alterations of membrane fluidity, modulation of AMPA (a subtype of glutmate) receptors, and increased brain adenosine triphosphate (ATP) levels (44–47). Piracetam is excreted unchanged in the urine. Lower doses are needed in elderly and renally impaired patients. Piracetam can inhibit platelet aggregation and should be discontinued before elective surgery. Use with Coumadin (warfarin) increases the risk of bleeding. Side effects include nervousness, irritability, headache, agitation, dizziness, GI effects, abnormal movements (e.g., chorea), and (very rarely) hepatotoxicity.

A large but methodologically limited literature suggests that piracetam can enhance cognition in animals and humans (47–51). Disorders for which piracetam may be beneficial include Alzheimer disease, autism, poststroke aphasia, dyslexia, and memory impairment associated with brain disorders (52–55). However, current evidence does not clearly support piracetam for treating patients with cognitive disorders (52, 56). Piracetam can improve epileptic and nonepileptic myoclonic disorders (57–58).

Ginkgo biloba

Ginkgo biloba is a tree whose seeds have been used for millennia in Chinese medicine. Leaf extracts are sold as dietary supplements with the main active ingredients flavonoid glycosides and ginkgolides. Ginkgolides are unique diterpenes with antioxidant effects, platelet activating factor inhibition, and circulatory enhancing effects (59). One extract of *Ginkgo biloba* (EGb) may exert potential cognitive and circulatory effects (60). *Ginkgo* extracts may improve memory function in Alzheimer disease, other dementias, and age-related memory impairment (59–60). A meta-analysis of 9 controlled trials in dementia found that the effect of EGb was superior to placebo in cognitive measures but not in activities of daily life (61). An analysis of 36 studies on cognitive benefits of *Ginkgo* and EGb found that there is no consistent evidence for efficacy in healthy adults or patients with dementia (62). Of 4 recent and adequately powered (i.e., have sufficient sample size, study duration, etc to statistically answer the question) studies, 3 found no difference between *Ginkgo* and placebo, while one found a large treatment effect. A double-blind controlled study found that 250 mg/d of *Ginkgo biloba* did not prevent dementia in elderly individuals or those with mild cognitive impairment (63). In summary, the data on the cognitive effects of *Ginkgo biloba* and EGb suggest that there may be small beneficial effects on cognition in some individuals, but in most, there is not functionally significant benefit.

Ginkgo has adverse event profiles similar to placebo (62–63). However, Ginkgo and other plant derivatives may increase the risk of bleeding in patients taking warfarin (64). People with epilepsy should be cautious of Ginkgo use. Ginkgo nuts as well as Ginkgo biloba extracts are temporally associated with seizures in patients without a prior history as well as in people with epilepsy (65–69). In at least one case, the seizure was fatal and was associated with subtherapeutic AED levels, suggesting possible induction of hepatic metabolism (69). Prospective data are needed to assess the potential beneficial and adverse effects of Ginkgo in people with epilepsy.

Caffeine

Caffeine is a xanthine alkaloid that primarily alters behavior as a nonselective antagonist of adenosine receptors (70). It also inhibits phosphodiesterase and prevents the inactivation of 2 intracellular second messengers: cyclic adenosine monophosphate and cyclic guanosine monophosphate. In humans, it is absorbed within 45 minutes and has a half-life of approximately 5 hours. Caffeine has potent effects on cardiovascular and brain function. It can increase alertness, performance, and, in some studies, memory (71). Caffeine improves performance in shift workers (72). Children and adults who consume low doses of caffeine showed increase alertness, yet a higher dose is needed to improve performance (73). Some studies show that caffeine may have a greater impact on improving cognitive performance and sustaining attention, while others show that caffeine is associated with declining function in the elderly (74). Caffeine can improve speed and accuracy of performance in cognitively demanding tasks (75). Caffeine use was not associated with increased risk of seizures or epilepsy in a large prospective study of women, although some case reports suggest that very high caffeine consumption can aggravate epilepsy in susceptible individuals (76–78).

Caffeine effects on the brain are controversial. Some admit to their effect on the brain, while others emphasize addictive and tolerance effects. Caffeine can help improve short-term concentration and facilitate learning as well as memory. Caffeine dilates the blood vessels in the brain when consumed in small amounts. In low doses, it increases alertness, but a high dose is needed to show improved performance. After consumption, it is rapidly distributed throughout the body and blocks actions of endogenous adenosine at adenosine A1 and A2, receptors resulting in different physiologic effects. The blockage is how caffeine can affect alertness and performance, since adenosine is closely involved in sleep regulation.

Antioxidant Therapy

There is a balance between the generation and elimination of reactive oxygen ions and peroxides. Excess reactive oxygen species can cause lipid peroxidation in neural membranes. However, there is a natural balance, and a certain level of oxidant activity may be beneficial. The role of vitamin E for general and neurologic health remains controversial since too much of a good thing can be bad (79–80). Medicine has yet to define the right amount of vitamin E consumption. Oxidative neuronal injury mediated by beta-amyloid may be an important cause of Alzheimer disease. Thus, antioxidants could theoretically prevent or slow the degeneration in Alzheimer disease. A 2-year RCT showed that the antioxidants selegiline (10 mg/d) and α-tocopherol (vitamin E, 2,000 IU/d) can retard decline in cognition and ability to perform activities of daily life and prolong survival in patients with moderate-severity Alzheimer disease (81). Patients treated with selegiline, α-tocopherol, or both improved in all clinical outcomes compared with those receiving placebo. There was no advantage of combined therapy versus either antioxidant alone. Further support comes from a meta-analysis of 15 studies showing that selegiline improves memory in Alzheimer disease (82). Consistent behavioral improvements were not demonstrated in this analysis. Other therapies such as estrogen replacement therapy in postmenopausal women and nonsteroidal antiinflammatory agents are of uncertain value in preventing or slowing the progression of Alzheimer disease. However, population-based studies reveal that individuals on these therapies have a lower rate of dementia (83).

Antioxidants may benefit brain functioning in many ways. Antioxidants protect the brain from oxidative damage. Recent studies suggest that vegetables help people retain their mental abilities longer and keep their brains younger. This may be because of vitamin E, folate, and antioxidant content in vegetables (84). The vegetables emphasized were often leafy green or cruciferous vegetables.

VITAMIN E

Vitamin E is a free radical–scavenging antioxidant that may help stabilize neural membrane phospholipids rich in polyunsaturated fatty acids. Vitamin E deficiency is rare and can cause a neurologic disorder of spinocerebellar degeneration, polyneuropathy, and pigmentary degeneration. Available data do not support the use of Vitamin E to improve cognitive function in patients with Alzheimer disease or in women at risk for cardiovascular disease (85–86). High-dose vitamin E may cause GI upset or impair clotting mechanisms, leading to easy bruising or bleeding. Vitamin E should be stopped at least 1 week before elective surgery. In one study, vitamin E supplementation did not improve seizure control (87). Institutionalized children with severe neurologic disability had nutritional deficiencies for vitamins E and D and other nutrients (88).

ISOFLAVONES

Isoflavones are naturally occurring compounds, found most often in beans, that have antioxidant properties. Many isoflavones (e.g., genistein and daidzein) are phytoestrogens, and this may account for the reduced the risk of some cancers (e.g., breast) with supplementation. In one controlled trial, isoflavones did not improve cognition (89).

Consumption of isoflavones, in the form of 50 mg of soy dietary supplements twice a day for 3 weeks, decreased a biomarker of DNA oxidation damage. Isoflavones are richest in soy products but can also be found in foods such as legumes. It is not overwhelming, but there is some evidence suggesting that isoflavones may protect the brain from cognitive decline.

Wong et al (90) found that the United Kingdom Joint Health believed that soy protein helps to reduce cholesterol, which may impact how the brain works. Another study looked mainly at the effects of soy on females during their cycle, since their estrogen levels constantly changed, and suggested that dietary phytoestrogens may have effects on cognitive function in females and that soy appeared to affect some cognitive processes (91).

POLYPHENOLICS

Polyphenolics are present in fruits and vegetables, with the highest concentrations in more darkly colored plants. These compounds have antioxidant and antiinflammatory properties. At high levels, they may retard and reverse elements of brain aging, such as dopamine decrease and other cognitive deficits.

Blueberries, blackberries, concord grapes, and strawberries contain high amounts of proanthocyanidins and anthocyanins. They are linked with improved cognitive function in animals and man, but data in humans are weakly supported by short open-label trials (92–93). Given the supportive animal data and safety of these fruits and phytochemicals, additional studies in both healthy and patient populations are warranted.

Polyphenolics in fruits and vegetables help brain functioning. The darker-colored fruits and vegetables tend to be high in phenolics, therefore possessing large antioxidant and inflammatory activity. At such levels, these effects can retard and reverse aspects of brain aging, such as dopamine release and other cognitive deficits. The polyphenols increase antioxidant and antiinflammatory levels. Such effects are particularly effective with dietary intake of berry fruit. A study was done on rats, where a 2% blackberry supplemented diet was proven effective in reversing age-related deficits and neural function. This diet helped improve motor performance on 3 tasks.

Polyphenolics positively affect brain signaling to enhance neural communication. Berries are also high in flavonoids, condensed and hydrolysable tannins, phenolic acids, and stillbenoids, among other substances, such as cyanidin-3-O-glucoside, which has the highest oxygen radial absorbance capacity among anthocyanins. Blackberries are very high in antiproliferative, antioxidant, and antiinflammatory activities, making them a great food for the brain. In one study proving the benefits of blackberries, rats were fed a 2% blackberry diet, and they were able to perform much better on behavioral tests than the control rats. Blackberry juice and its main anthocyanin component, cyanidin-3-O-glucoside may have a protective effect against free radical–medicated endothelial dysfunction and vascular disorders. Blackberries, like blueberries, may exert their protective effects directly through alterations in cell signaling to improve or increase neuronal communication, calcium buffering ability, neuroprotective stress shock proteins, plasticity, and stress signaling pathways (94). The study found that the blueberry diet improved spatial working memory in older rats, and changes were regulated by the cyclic adenosine monophosphate response element binding and brain-derived neurotropic factor pathway in the hippocampus. Anthocyanins, which are found in blueberries and blackberries, enter the brain and may improve cognitive function.

ω-3 FATTY ACIDS

ω-3 fatty acids are unsaturated fats that are part of a healthy diet. These are essential nutrients since the body cannot synthesize them, and they must be obtained from the diet. Two long-chain ω-3 fatty acids, docosahexaenoic acid (DHA) and eicosapentaenoic acid (EPA), are associated most strongly with reduced cardiovascular risk but also with reduced risk of prostate and breast cancer (95–96). European investigators failed to find significant benefits for Alzheimer disease with ω-3 fatty acid supplementation (97). A Norwegian study found that long-chain ω-3 fatty acid (DHA) supplementation during pregnancy and lactation was associated with higher cognitive test scores at age 4 years (98).

SELEGILINE

Selegiline is an irreversible selective monoamine oxidase type B (MAO-B) inhibitor that blocks presynaptic reuptake of catecholamines and presynaptic dopamine autoreceptors, thereby enhancing dopaminergic activity (99). It was introduced as an adjunctive therapy in Parkinson disease with postulated neuroprotective effects mediated by slowing striatal dopamine metabolism. Selegiline can delay the need to initiate levodopa therapy and decrease the dosages required; it may improve memory and motor functions (100). The standard dose is 5 mg twice daily. Selegiline may improve cognitive function, but it did not improve cognition in a 6-month trial in patients with HIV (101). Selegiline did increase attention in children with the inattentive subtype of ADD (14). Selegiline is metabolized in the liver into active metabolites. Doses higher than 10 mg/d also inhibit MAO-A. The peripheral side effects are milder than those of nonspecific MAO inhibitors and include nausea, dizziness, anorexia, headache, hypotension, and increased libido. Central nervous system side effects include insomnia, anxiety, agitation, psychosis, hallucinations, confusion, and dyskinesias. Hypertensive crisis induced with tyramine-rich foods is less with selegiline than with other MAO inhibitors, especially at lower doses. Selegiline should be used cautiously with serotonin reuptake inhibitors, tricyclic antidepressants, or meperidine (opiates).

PHOSPHATIDYLSERINE

Phosphatidylserine is an important component of neuronal membranes, involved in ATP production, ion homeostasis, and synaptic function. Data from small and uncontrolled studies suggest a potential role of phosphatidylserine for memory, learning, concentration, word retrieval, and stress tolerance in dementia, ADD, and other clinical groups (102). However, subsequent studies failed to show any beneficial effects (103). Recommended doses of phosphatidylserine range between 100 mg/d in children and 200 to 600 mg/d in adults to improve cognition or mood. Oral phosphatidylserine and γ-aminobutyric acid had no effect on the photoconvulsive response in patients with generalized epilepsy (104).

ACETYL-L-CARNITINE

Acetyl-L-carnitine is a metabolic cofactor in mitochondria that transports fatty acids during their oxidation to generate energy. It also provides acetyl groups for ACh synthesis. Acetyl-L-carnitine crosses the blood-brain barrier more efficiently than L-carnitine. The largest trial of acetyl-L-carnitine found no benefit for patients with Alzheimer disease (105). A subsequent subgroup analysis found that acetyl-L-carnitine may slow the progression of dementia in younger patients (106). Several smaller studies found acetyl-L-carnitine improved cognitive and behavioral function in ex-alcoholics (107). Relatively high doses of acetyl-L-carnitine (1,500–2,000 mg/d) were used in most studies, and side effects included intense dreams. Intracerebral injection of acetyl-L-carnitine into rats induced immediate interictal and ictal epileptic changes, probably related to muscarinic agonism (108).

BACOPA

Bacopa (*Bacopa monnieri*, aka water hyssop) has been used in India as an Ayurvedic (traditional) herbal to enhance cognition and treat psychiatric disorders and epilepsy (109). The active ingredients, derived from the leaves, are steroidal saponins, including the bacosides. Uncontrolled trials in India found that 12 g/d of the dried plant for 4 weeks improved concentration, immediate memory, and anxiety (110). In the United States, 300 mg of *B monnieri* extract improved memory and Stroop test scores in healthy elderly adults without significant side effects (111). In rats, *B monnieri* extract was protective against glutamate-mediated excitotoxicity during seizures and cognitive damage occurring in association with pilocarpine-induced seizures (112).

VINPOCETINE

Vinpocetine is an alkaloid derived from the lesser periwinkle (*Vinca minor*). It is a free radical scavenger and a potent vasodilator, directly relaxing vascular smooth muscle (47, 113). Vinpocetine enhances cerebral blood flow in patients with stroke (114) and decreases platelet and red blood cell aggregation and blood viscosity (114–115). Vinpocetine improved cognition in several studies of patients with vascular dementia and poststroke cognitive problems (47, 113, 116–117). An RCT in patients with Alzheimer disease found that vinpocetine was safe but ineffective (118). Antiepileptic effects have been suggested but not proven (119). Doses of 15 to 45 mg/d were used in most studies. Side effects include flushing, rash, and nausea.

TYROSINE

Tyrosine is an amino acid and the precursor for the neurotansmitters dopamine, norepinephrine, and epinephrine. Although there is little or no evidence that tyrosine has benefits in normal conditions, supplemental tyrosine helped to prevent memory loss, headaches, and lightheadedness in soldiers exposed to high altitudes or prolonged cold (120–123).

B VITAMINS

Although commonly promoted in supplements as "brain food," there is little evidence that B vitamins improve cognitive function. The observation that levels of homocysteine, a sulfur-containing amino acid involved in essential metabolic pathways such as methylation, are elevated in neuropsychiatric disorders led to the concept that vitamin B_{12} or folate deficiencies may cause these disorders. Neither healthy nor cognitively impaired individuals appear to benefit from B vitamin supplements, including various combinations that include folic acid as well as vitamin B_{12} injections (124–125). Rarely, vitamin B_6 deficiency causes severe neonatal seizures that often only respond to vitamin B_6 supplementation (126).

FATIGUE

Fatigue is common among people with epilepsy and is often a result of AEDs and seizures. Fatigue can manifest as lack of energy, tiredness, premature exhaustion from mental or physical activity, and an aversion to effort. Fatigue is commonly overlooked since all of us grow familiar with our environment. Tolerance develops to both pleasurable and adverse settings. Initiation of a sedating AED leads to complaints of fatigue. After weeks and months, the declining rates and severity of fatigue are assumed to reflect tolerance to the adverse effect of the AED. However, it may be equally probable that patients grow used to the side effect but that the side effects persist. Consider the following case of ours:

> A 33-year-old woman with medically refractory epilepsy was evaluated for surgical therapy. She denied any adverse effects of her AEDs. Following video electroencephalographic monitoring, she was tapered off of phenobarbital and started on lamotrigine. Shortly after completion of the conversion, her employer contacted the physician to report a dramatic improvement in the patient's level of energy, mental processing speed, and memory. The side effects were there, but she had grown accustomed to them.

Treatment for fatigue includes reduction or elimination of sedating medications, therapy for comorbid mood disorders, education about energy conservation techniques, medications (amantadine, modafinil, armodafinil and stimulants), exercise, and stress management techniques (127). We lack systematic trials of drugs to improve fatigue in people with epilepsy.

Nootropic drugs are used primarily to treat people with cognitive difficulties such as Alzheimer disease, Parkinson disease, and ADHD. However, use is more widespread, including potential abuse by students (128). These drugs have a variety of human enhancement applications as well and are marketed heavily on the Internet. Nevertheless, intense marketing may not correlate with efficacy; while scientific studies support some of the claimed benefits, it is worth noting that many of the claims attributed to most nootropics have not been formally tested.

Modafinil and armodafinil can increase productivity, but long-term effects have not been assessed in healthy individuals (129). They can reduce excessive daytime somnolence after traumatic brain injury (130). Stimulants such as methylphenidate are being used on college campuses and by an increasingly younger group (129). One survey found that 7% of students had used stimulants for a cognitive edge in the past year, and on some campuses, the number is as high as 25% (131).

SEROTONERGICS

Serotonin is a neurotransmitter with various effects on mood and possible effects on neurogenesis. Serotonergics are substances that affect the neurotransmitter serotonin or the components of the nervous system that use serotonin. Serotonergic nootropics include serotonin precursors and cofactors and serotonin reuptake inhibitors (Table 10.2).

Table 10.2   Serotonergics

5-HTP	Precursor
Tryptophan	Essential amino acid precursor
SSRIs	Class of antidepressants that increase serotonin levels by inhibiting its reuptake
	Have been shown to promote neurogenesis in hippocampus
Kanna	Herb with antidepressant properties
	Shown to act as a potent SSRI
Tianeptine	Paradoxical antidepressant
	Improves mood and reduces anxiety

Abbreviations: 5-HTP, 5-hydroxytryptophan; SSRI, selective serotonin reuptake inhibitor.

Table 10.3 Adaptogenic Drug and Substances

β-blockers	Anxiolytic
Lemon balm	Adaptogen properties; shown to possess GABA transaminase inhibitor properties
Passion flower	Possible MAOI and neurotransmitter reuptake activity
Rhodiola rosea	Adaptogen properties; possible MAOI activity
St. John's wort	Herbal SSRI approved (in Europe) to treat mild depression
Ginseng (including Siberian ginseng)	Adaptogen properties
Sutherlandia frutescens	Possible antiinflammatory effects; reduces pain
Kava	Anxiolytic herb
Tea	Many different adaptogens
Theanine	GABAergic activity; produces relaxation and increases brain serotonin and dopamine levels
Grape seed extract	Some efficacy in reduction of bodily stress
Adafenoxate	Possible anxiolytic
Valerian	Possible anxiolytic via GABA-A receptor agonism
Butea frondosa	Possible anxiolytic effect
Gotu kola	Adaptogen properties; anxiolytic
Foti	Adaptogen properties; possible MAOI activity
Berberine	Alkaloid, found in various herbs; antidepressant properties; acts as sigma receptor agonist; acts as mild tyrosine hydroxylase inhibitor

Abbreviations: GABA, γ-aminobutyric acid; MAOI, monoamine oxidase inhibitor; SSRI, selective serotonin reuptake inhibitor.

Stress, depression, and depressed mood negatively affect cognitive performance. It is reasoned that counteracting and preventing depression and stress may be an effective nootropic strategy. The term *adaptogenic* applies to most herbal antistress claims.

Table 10.3 summarizes adaptogenic drugs and substances.

BLOOD FLOW, METABOLIC FUNCTION, AND ANTIOXIDANTS

Brain function is dependent on many basic processes, such as the use of ATP, removal of waste, and intake of new materials. Improving blood flow or altering these processes can benefit brain function. Vasodilators and other drugs and

Table 10.4 Vasodilators and Substances that may Affect Brain Metabolism

Blessed thistle	Increases blood circulation; improves memory
Creatine	Protects ATP during transport
Lipoic acid	Improves oxygen use and antioxidant recycling; possibly improves memory
Pyritinol	Drug; similar to B vitamin pyridoxine
Picamilon	Improves GABA activity and blood flow
Ginkgo biloba	Vasodilator; shown to act as GABA-A receptor negative allosteric modulator and GABA-A-rho receptor antagonist (formerly known as GABA-C receptors)
Vinpocetine	Vasodilator; increases brain metabolism; inhibits voltage-sensitive Na+ channels
Reserpine	May inhibit VMAT and temporarily deplete monoamines (serotonin, dopamine, norepinephrine), preventing monoamine activity in synapse; induces or exacerbates depressive symptoms

Abbreviations: ATP, adenosine triphosphate; GABA, γ-aminobutyric acid; VMAT, vesicular monoamine transporter.

substances with potential effects on brain metabolism are mentioned in Table 10.4. Drugs that have antioxidant effects and may protect the brain from other stressors could potentially improve brain functions, but these benefits on brain functions are unproven. Selected ones are summarized in Table 10.5.

Antioxidants are frequently used to prevent oxidative stress but do not improve brain function if that is their only activity (Table 10.5).

Table 10.5 Antioxidants and Neuroprotectors

Coenzyme Q10	Antioxidant; increases mitochondria oxygen use
Idebenone	Antioxidant
Melatonin	Antioxidant
Glutathione	Chief antioxidant
Acetylcarnitine (acetyl-L-carnitine arginate or hydrochloride)	Neuroprotective
Citicoline (cytidine 5-diphosphocholine)	Neuroprotective

(continued)

Table 10.5   Antioxidants and Neuroprotectors (*continued*)

Inositol	Implicated in memory function; deficit linked to some psychiatric illnesses; possibly efficacious in patients with OCD
Antiepileptic drugs	Inhibit seizure-related brain malfunction if a person has AEDs
Phosphatidylserine	Possible membrane stabilizer
Lion's mane mushroom	Stimulated myelination in an in vitro experiment (135) and stimulated nerve growth factor in an in vitro experiment with human astrocytoma cells (136); also improved cognitive ability in a double-blind, parallel-group, placebo-controlled trial (137)
SAM-e	Possibly involved in cellular regeneration (fuels DNA methylation); also involved with the biosynthesis of dopamine and serotonin (138)
Acetylcysteine (L-cysteine)	Precursor to antioxidant glutathione
Apoaequorin (calcium-binding protein; CaBP, Prevagen®)	Neuroprotective
Dopamine enhancers	Dopamine is an antioxidant and can enhance dendrite extension

Abbreviations: CaBP, calcium-binding protein; OCD, obsessive-compulsive disorder; SAM-e, S-adenosyl methionine.

DIETARY NOOTROPICS

Diet can potentially affect cognition and brain function, as there are many necessary nutrients that must be consumed. However, other substances have been linked to certain benefits and may be predominant in certain foods. Studies link vitamin B_1, vitamin B_{12}, ω-3, antioxidants, protein, and iron to brain function. It is crucial to obtain the nutrients that increase cognitive function directly as well as those that affect how those nutrients are absorbed and used in the body.

Vitamin B_1, thiamin, aids nerve cell function and helps the body convert food, specifically carbohydrates, into glucose. Glucose is what the brain runs off of, making it crucial for the brain. Foods containing vitamin B_1 include whole grains, rice, wheat germ, bran, and organ meats. Vitamin B_{12}, cobalamin, is used to make neurotransmitters. It also maintains the nervous system by helping to metabolize fatty acids, which are essential for the maintenance of myelin, which surrounds nerves. Vitamin B_{12} is found primarily in animal products, but it may also be found in soy products, eggs, seaweed, and algae. Low amounts of vitamin B_{12} with normal folate levels may cause cognitive impairment and anemia, while high amounts of folate and normal vitamin B_{12} levels may improve cognitive function (132).

Adult brains use amino acids, which are typically found in protein-rich food, for the production of enzymes that transport molecules, structural material, and neurotransmitters, along with other essential molecules. Some of the amino acids include tyrosine and phenylalanine, which help to produce the hormone epinephrine and neurotransmitter dopamine. These 2 hormones help create alertness. Therefore, it is suggested to eat low-carbohydrates but high-protein meals, so people are more alert and attentive. However, too much protein can have a negative effect as well since they are not complete source of nutrients. Tryptophan, a precursor to the neurotransmitter serotonin, helps to stabilize mood and may also influence the cognitive process, specifically learning and memory. There have been both human and rat studies that have indicated a deficit in long-term memory and information processing due to tryptophan depletion, and other studies show how tryptophan helps to improve decision making. Although carbohydrates do not contain tryptophan, they may help to push tryptophan into the brain by triggering the release of insulin. Insulin stimulates muscles to take up competing amino acids. Even calcium, which typically comes in many foods with protein, helps regulate nerve impulse transmission (133). Another

Table 10.6   Possible Nootropics, Unknown Enhancement

Nootropics with proven or purported benefits	
Bacopa monnieri	Adaptogenic properties
	May enhance memory and concentration (139)
	Folk use in Ayurvedic medicine purports "enhancement of curiosity"
Brahmi rasayana	May improve learning and memory in mice (140)
Fipexide	Possible benefits for dementia
Gerovital H3	Antiaging mixture; most effects disproven but some mind enhancement possible
Sulbutiamine	Fat-soluble vitamin B_1 derivative; possible memory improvement
Royal jelly	Can increase brain cell growth in cell experiments; improbable *in vivo*
Curcumin	Significant in vitro activity, but *in vivo* activity is limited by low bioavailability
Other nootropics (These substances have been linked to better cognitive function but may not be the cause)	
Moderate use of alcohol	Moderate drinkers may have better cognition function than both abstainers and heavy drinkers (141–145)

important neurotransmitters is serotonin. Acetylcholine is essential in memory formation and maintenance. It is found in egg yolks, soy, nuts, seeds and organ meats. Creation and use of ACh is crucial for memory. Serotonin helps with sleep regulation and anxiety reduction. It is manufactured from tryptophan (134).

Iron is also important for staying mentally sharp. Iron helps create hemoglobin, an iron containing protein in red blood cells, which transports oxygen to the brain. Oxygen in the brain is vital since it helps to metabolize glucose. Insufficient iron in the diet of a child can lead to impaired brain development and deficits in speech, math, and reading skills. Women of reproductive age need the most iron and therefore may be more likely to end up with a deficiency. Those with sufficient iron in their blood have been proven to perform better on cognitive tests than those who were iron deficient.

POSSIBLE NOOTROPICS WITH UNKNOWN MECHANISMS

Other agents purported to have nootropic effects but that do not (yet) have attributable mechanisms or clinically significant effects are summarized in Table 10.6.

REFERENCES

1. Symonds C. Discussion. *Proc R Soc Med*. 1962;55:314–315.
2. Gallagher AL, Chiat S. Evaluation of speech and language therapy interventions for preschool children with specific language impairment: a comparison of outcomes following specialist intensive, nursery-based and no intervention. *Int J Lang Commun Disord*. 2009;44:616–638.
3. Meikle M, Wechsler E, Tupper A, Benenson M, Butler J, Mulhall D, Stern G. Comparative trial of volunteer and professional treatments of dysphasia after stroke. *Br Med J*. 1979;2:87–89.
4. Bakheit AM, Shaw S, Barrett L, et al. A prospective, randomized, parallel group, controlled study of the effect of intensity of speech and language therapy on early recovery from poststroke aphasia. *Clin Rehabil*. 2007;21(10):885–94.
5. Cicerone KD, Dahlberg C, Kalmar K, et al. Evidence-based cognitive rehabilitation: Recommendations for clinical practice. *Arch Phys Med Rehabil*. 2000;81:1596–1615.
6. Unverzagt FW, Smith DM, Rebok GW, et al. The Indiana Alzheimer Disease Center's Symposium on mild cognitive impairment. Cognitive training in older adults: lessons from the ACTIVE Study. *Curr Alzheimer Res*. 2009;6:375–383.
7. Giurgea C. Vers une pharmacologie de l'active integrative du cerveau: tentative du concept nootrope en psychopharmacologie. *Actual Pharmacol (Paris)*. 1972;25:115–156.
8. Solanto MV, Marks DJ, Wasserstein J, et al. Efficacy of meta-cognitive therapy for adult ADHD. *Am J Psychiatry*. 2010;167:958–956.
9. Pfiffner LJ, Yee Mikami A, Huang-Pollock C, Easterlin B, Zalecki C, McBurnett K. A randomized, controlled trial of integrated home-school behavioral treatment for ADHD, predominantly inattentive type. *J Am Acad Child Adolesc Psychiatry*. 2007;46:1041–1050.
10. Karpouzis F, Bonello R, Pollard H. Chiropractic care for paediatric and adolescent attention-deficit/hyperactivity disorder: a systematic review. *Chiropr Osteopat*. 2010;18:13.

11. Dell'Agnello G, Maschietto D, Bravaccio C, et al. Atomoxetine hydrochloride in the treatment of children and adolescents with attention-deficit/hyperactivity disorder and comorbid oppositional defiant disorder: a placebo-controlled Italian study. *Eur Neuropsychopharmacol.* 2009;19:822–834.

12. Bangs ME, Hazell P, Danckaerts M, et al. Atomoxetine for the treatment of attention-deficit/hyperactivity disorder and oppositional defiant disorder. *Pediatrics.* 2008;121: e314–e320.

13. Turner DC, Clark L, Dowson J, Robbins TW, Sahakian BJ. Modafinil improves cognition and response inhibition in adult attention-deficit/hyperactivity disorder. *Biol Psychiatry.* 2004;55:1031–1040.

14. Rubinstein S, Malone MA, Roberts W, Logan WJ. Placebo-controlled study examining effects of selegiline in children with attention-deficit/hyperactivity disorder. *J Child Adolesc Psychopharmacol.* 2006;16:404–415.

15. Potter AS, Newhouse PA. Acute nicotine improves cognitive deficits in young adults with attention-deficit/hyperactivity disorder. *Pharmacol Biochem Behav.* 2008;88:407–417.

16. Wernicke JF, Holdridge KC, Jin L, et al. Seizure risk in patients with attention-deficit-hyperactivity disorder treated with atomoxetine. *Dev Med Child Neurol.* 2007;49:498–502.

17. Hamoda HM, Guild DJ, Gumlak S, Travers BH, Gonzalez-Heydrich J. Association between attention-deficit/hyperactivity disorder and epilepsy in pediatric populations. *Expert Rev Neurother.* 2009;9:1747–1754.

18. Hermann B, Jones J, Dabbs K, et al. The frequency, complications and aetiology of ADHD in new onset paediatric epilepsy. *Brain.* 2007;130:3135–3148.

19. Borgatti R, Piccinelli P, Montirosso R, et al. Study of attentional processes in children with idiopathic epilepsy by Conners' continuous performance test. *J Child Neurol.* 2004;19: 509–515.

20. Hesdorffer DC, Ludvigsson P, Olafsson E, Gudundsson G, Kjartansson O, Hauser WA. ADHD as a risk factor for incident unprovoked seizures and epilepsy in children. *Arch Gen Psychiatry.* 2004;61:731–736.

21. Davis SM, Katusic SK, Barbaresi WJ, et al. Epilepsy in children with attention-deficit/hyperactivity disorder. *Pediatr Neurol.* 2010;42:325–330.

22. Parisi P, Moavero R, Verrotti A, Curatolo P. Attention deficit hyperactivity disorder in children with epilepsy. *Brain Dev.* 2010;32:10–16.

23. Baptista-Neto L, Dodds A, Rao S, Whitney J, Torres A, Gonzalez-Heydrich J. An expert opinion on methylphenidate treatment for attention deficit hyperactivity disorder in pediatric patients with epilepsy. *Expert Opin Investig Drugs.* 2008;17:77–84.

24. *Physicians' Desk Reference.* Toronto, Ontario: Thomson Corp; 2011.

25. Tan M, Appleton R. Attention deficit and hyperactivity disorder, methylphenidate and epilepsy. *Arch Dis Child.* 2005;90:57–59.

26. Feldman H, Crumrine P, Handen BL, Alvin R, Teodori J. Methylphenidate in children with seizures and attention-deficit disorder. *Am J Dis Child.* 1989;143:1081–1086.

27. Van der Feltz-Cornelis CM, Aldenkamp AP. Effectiveness and safety of methylphenidate in adult attention deficit hyperactivity disorder in patients with epilepsy: an open treatment trial. *Epilepsy Behav.* 2006;8:659–662.

28. Torres AR, Whitney J, Gonzalez-Heydrich J. Attention-deficit/hyperactivity disorder in pediatric patients with epilepsy: review of pharmacological treatment. *Epilepsy Behav.* 2008;12:217–233.

29. Gross-Tsur V, Manor O, van der Meere J, Joseph A, Shalev RS. Epilepsy and attention deficit hyperactivity disorder: is methylphenidate safe and effective? *J Pediatr.* 1997;130:670–674.

30. McAfee AT, Holdridge KC, Johannes CB, Hornbuckle K, Walker AM. The effect of pharmacotherapy for attention deficit hyperactivity disorder on risk of seizures in pediatric patients as assessed in an insurance claims database. *Curr Drug Saf.* 2008;3:123–131.

31. Muir VJ, Perry CM. Guanfacine extended-release: in attention deficit hyperactivity disorder. *Drugs*. 2010;70:1693–1702.
32. Swartz BE, McDonald CR, Patel A, Torgersen D. The effects of guanfacine on working memory performance in patients with localization-related epilepsy and healthy controls. *Clin Neuropharmacol*. 2008;31:251–260.
33. Lovera JF, Frohman E, Brown TR, et al. Memantine for cognitive impairment in multiple sclerosis: a randomized placebo-controlled trial. *Mult Scler*. 2010;16:715–723.
34. Knapp MJ, Knopman DS, Soloman PR, Pendlebury WW, Davis CS, Gracon SI. A 30-week randomized controlled trial of high-dose tacrine in patients with Alzheimer's disease. *JAMA*. 1994;271:985–991.
35. Maltby N, Broe GA, Creasey H, Jorm AF, Christensen H, Brooks WS. Efficacy of tacrine and lecithin in mild to moderate Alzheimer's disease: double blind trial. *Br Med J*. 1994;271:992–998.
36. Fisher RS, Bortz JJ, Blum DE, Duncan B, Burke H. A pilot study of donepezil for memory problems in epilepsy. *Epilepsy Behav*. 2001;2:330–334.
37. Masanic CA, Bayley MT, VanReekum R, Simard M. Open-label study of donepezil in traumatic brain injury. *Arch Phys Med Rehabil*. 2001;82:896–901.
38. Lu PH, Edland SD, Teng E, et al. Donepezil delays progression to AD in MCI subjects with depressive symptoms. *Neurology*. 2009;72:2115–2121.
39. [NICE] National Institute for Health and Clinical Excellence. *Donepezil, Galantamine, Rivastigmine (Review) and Memantine for the Treatment of Alzheimer's Disease (Amended): Nice Technology Appraisal Guidance of 111 (Amended)*. London, England: National Health Service; 2007.
40. Areosa Sastre A, Sherriff F, McShane R. Memantine for dementia. *The Cochrane Database Syst Rev*. 2006;1:CD003154.
41. Atri A, Shaughnessy L, Locascio J, Growdon J. Long-term course and effectiveness of combination therapy in Alzheimer disease. *Alzheimer Dis Assoc Disord*. 2008;22:209–221.
42. Lopez OL, Becker JT, Wahed AS, et al. Long-term effects of the concomitant use of memantine with cholinesterase inhibition in Alzheimer disease. *J Neurol Neurosurg Psychiatry*. 2009;80:600–607.
43. Malykh AG, Sadaie MR. Piracetam and piracetam-like drugs: from basic science to novel clinical applications to CNS disorders. *Drugs*. 2010;70:287–312.
44. Eckert GP, Cairns NJ, Muller WE. Piracetam reverses hippocampal membrane alterations in Alzheimer's disease. *J Neural Transm*. 1999;106:757–761.
45. Muller WE, Eckert GP, Eckert A. Piracetam: novelty in a unique mode of action. *Pharmacopsychiatry*. 1999;32:2–9.
46. Ahmed A, Oswald R. Piracetam defines a new binding site for allosteric modulators of r-amino-3-hydroxy-5-methyl-4-isoxazole-proprionic acid (AMPA) receptors. *J Med Chem*. 2010;53:2197–2203.
47. Nicholson CD. Pharmacology of nootropics and metabolically active compounds in relation to their use in dementia. *Psychopharmacology (Berl)*. 1990;101:147–159.
48. Nicholson CD. Nootropics and metabolically active compounds in Alzheimer's disease. *Biochem Soc Trans*. 1989;17:83–85.
49. Flynn BL. Pharmacologic management of Alzheimer disease, part I: hormonal and emerging investigational drug therapies. *Ann Pharmacother*. 1999;33:178–187.
50. Noble S, Benfield P. Piracetam. *CNS Drugs*. 1998;9:497–511.
51. Poeck K. Piracetam treatment in post-stroke aphasia. *CNS Drugs*. 1998;suppl 1:51–56.
52. Flicker L, Grimely Evans G. Piracetam for dementia or cognitive impairment. *Cochrane Database Syst Rev*. 2001;2:CD001011.
53. Paczyniski M. Piracetam: A novel therapy for autism? *J Autism Dev Discord*. 1997;27:628–630.

54. Huber W, Willmes K, Poeck K, van Vleymen B, Deberdt W. Piracetam as an adjuvant to language therapy for aphasia: a randomized double-blind placebo-controlled pilot study. *Arch Phys Med Rehabil.* 1997;78:245–250.

55. Wilsher CR, Bennett D, Chase CH, et al. Piracetam and dyslexia: effects on reading tests. *J Clin Psychopharmacol.* 1987;7:230–237.

56. Ackerman PT, Dykman RA, Holloway C, Paal NP, Gocio MY. A trial of piracetam in two subgroups of students with dyslexia enrolled in summer tutoring. *J Learn Disabil.* 1991;24:542–549.

57. Obeso JA, Artieda J, Quinn N, Rothwell JC, Luquin MR, Vaamonde J. Piracetam in the treatment of different types of myoclonus. *Clin Neuropharmacol.* 1988;11:529–536.

58. Fedi M, Reutens D, Dubeau F, Andermann E, D'Agostino D, Andermann F. Long-term efficacy and safety of piracetam in the treatment of progressive myoclonus epilepsy. *Arch Neurol.* 2001;58:781–786.

59. McKenna DJ, Jones K, Hughes K. Efficacy, safety, and use of *Ginkgo biloba* in clinical and preclinical applications. *Altern Ther Health Med.* 2001;7:88–90.

60. DeFeudis FV, Drieu K. *Ginkgo biloba* extract (EGb 761) and CNS functions: basic studies and clinical applications. *Curr Drug Targets.* 2000;1:25–58.

61. Weinmann S, Roll S, Schwarzbach C, Vauth C, Willich SN. Effects of *Gingko biloba* in dementia: systematic review and meta-analysis. *BMC Geriatr.* 2010;10:14.

62. Birks J, Grimley Evans J. *Ginkgo biloba* for cognitive impairment and dementia. *Cochrane Database Syst Rev.* 2009;1CD003120.

63. Dekosky ST, Williamson JD, Fitzpatrick AL, et al. *Ginkgo biloba* for prevention of dementia: a randomized controlled trial. *JAMA.* 2008;300:2253–2262.

64. Heck AM, DeWitt BA, Lukes AL. Potential interactions between alternative therapies and warfarin. *Am J Health Syst Pharm.* 2000;57:1221–1227.

65. Granger AS. *Ginkgo biloba* precipitating epileptic seizures. *Age Ageing.* 2001;30:523–525.

66. Miwa H, Iijima M, Tanaka S, Mizuno Y. Generalized convulsions after consuming a large amount of gingko nuts. *Epilepsia.* 2001;42:280–281.

67. Gregory PJ. Seizure associated with *Ginkgo biloba*? *Ann Intern Med.* 2001;134:344.

68. Haller CA, Meier KH, Olson KR. Seizures reported in association with use of dietary supplements. *Clin Toxicol (Phila).* 2005;43:23–30.

69. Kupiec T, Raj V. Fatal seizures due to potential herb-drug interactions with *Ginkgo biloba*. *J Anal Toxicol.* 2005;29:755–758.

70. Fisone G, Borgkvist A, Usiello A. Caffeine as a psychomotor stimulant: mechanism of action. *Cell Mol Life Sci.* 2004;61:857–872.

71. Childs E, de Wit H. Subjective, behavioral, and physiological effects of acute caffeine in light, nondependent caffeine users. *Psychopharmacology.* 2006;185:514–523.

72. Ker K, Edwards PJ, Felix LM, Blackhall K, Roberts I. Caffeine for the prevention of injuries and errors in shift workers. *Cochrane Database Syst Rev.* 2010;5:CD008508.

73. Kiefer I. Brain food. *Sci Am Mind.* 2007;18:58–63.

74. Lesk VE, Honey TE, de Jager CA. The effect of recent consumption of caffeine-containing foodstuffs on neuropsychological tests in the elderly. *Dement Geriatr Cogn Disord.* 2009;27:322–328.

75. Owen GN, Parnell H, De Bruin EA, Rycroft JA. The combined effects of L-theanine and caffeine on cognitive performance and mood. *Nutr Neurosci.* 2008;11:193–198.

76. Dworetzky BA, Bromfield EB, Townsend MK, Kang JH. A prospective study of smoking, caffeine, and alcohol as risk factors for seizures or epilepsy in young adult women: data from Nurses' Health Study II. *Epilepsia.* 2010;51:198–205.

77. Bonilha L, Li LM. Heavy coffee drinking and epilepsy. *Seizure.* 2004;13:284–285.

78. Kaufman KR, Sachdeo RC. Caffeinated beverages and decreased seizure control. *Seizure.* 2003;12:519–521.

79. Traber MG, Frei B, Beckman JS. Vitamin E revisited: do new data validate benefits for chronic disease prevention? *Curr Opin Lipidol.* 2008;19:30–38.
80. Mudway IS, Behndig AF, Helleday R, et al. Vitamin supplementation does not protect against symptoms in ozone-responsive subjects. *Free Radic Biol Med.* 2006;40:1702–1712.
81. Sano M, Ernesto C, Thomas RG, et al. A controlled trial of selegiline, alpha-tocopherol, or both as treatment for Alzheimer's disease. The Alzheimer's Disease Cooperative Study. *N Engl J Med.* 1997;336:1216–1222.
82. Birks J, Flicker L. Selegiline for Alzheimer's disease. *Cochrane Database Syst Rev.* 2000;2:CD000442.
83. Cummings JL. Treatment of Alzheimer's disease. *Clin Cornerstone.* 2001;3:27–39.
84. Nurk E, Refsum H, Drevon CA, et al. Cognitive performance among the elderly in relation to the intake of plant foods. The Hordaland Health Study. *Br J Nutr.* 2010;104(8): 1190–1201.
85. Nurk E, Refsum H, Drevon CA, et al. Vitamin E paradox in Alzheimer's disease: it does not prevent loss of cognition and may even be detrimental. *J Alzheimers Dis.* 2009;17: 143–149.
86. Kang JH, Cook NR, Manson JE, Buring JE, Albert CM, Grodstein F. Vitamin E, vitamin C, beta carotene, and cognitive function among women with or at risk of cardiovascular disease: the Women's Antioxidant and Cardiovascular Study. *Circulation.* 2009;119: 2772–2780.
87. Raju GB, Behari M, Prasad K, Ahuja GK. Randomized, double-blind, placebo-controlled, clinical trial of D-alpha-tocopherol (vitamin E) as add-on therapy in uncontrolled epilepsy. *Epilepsia.* 1994;35:368–372.
88. Hals J, Ek J, Svalastog AG, Nilsen H. Studies on nutrition in severely neurologically disabled children in an institution. *Acta Paediatr.* 1996;85:1469–1475.
89. Ho SC, Chan AS, Ho YP, et al. Effects of soy isoflavone supplementation on cognitive function in Chinese postmenopausal women: a double-blind, randomized, controlled trial. *Menopause.* 2007;14:489–499.
90. Wong MC, Emery PC, Preedy VR, Wiseman H. Health benefits of isoflavones in functional foods? Proteomic and metabonomic advances. *Inflammopharmacology.* 2008;16:235–239.
91. Zhao L, Brinton RD. WHI and WHIMS follow-up and human studies of soy isoflavones on cognition. *Expert Rev Neurother.* 2007;7:1549–1564.
92. Joseph J, Cole G, Head E, Ingram D. Nutrition, brain aging, and neurodegeneration. *J Neurosci.* 2009;29:12795–12801.
93. Krikorian R, Shidler MD, Nash TA, et al. Blueberry supplementation improves memory in older adults. *J Agric Food Chem.* 2010;58(7):3996–4000.
94. Beattie J, Crozier A, Duthie GG. Potential health benefits of berries. *Curr Nutr Food Sci.* 2005;1:71–86.
95. Marchioli R, Barzi F, Bomba E, et al. Early protection against sudden death by n-3 polyunsaturated fatty acids after myocardial infarction: time-course analysis of the results of the GISSI-Prevenzione. *Circulation.* 2002;105:1897–1903.
96. Berquin IM, Edwards IJ, Chen YQ. Multi-targeted therapy of cancer by omega-3 fatty acids. *Cancer Lett.* 2008;269:363–377.
97. Cederholm T, Palmblad J. Are omega-3 fatty acids options for prevention and treatment of cognitive decline and dementia? *Curr Opin Clin Nutr Metab Care.* 2010;13:150–155.
98. Helland IB, Smith L, Saarem K, Saugstad OD, Drevon CA. Maternal supplementation with very-long-chain n-3 fatty acids during pregnancy and lactation augments children's IQ at 4 years of age. *Pediatrics.* 2003;111:e39–e44.
99. Olanow CW. MAO-B inhibitors in Parkinson's disease. *Adv Neurol.* 1993;60:666–671.
100. Dixit SN, Behari M, Ahuja GK. Effect of selegiline on cognitive functions in Parkinson's disease. *J Assoc Physicians India.* 1999;47:784–786.

101. Evans SR, Yeh TM, Sacktor N, et al. Selegiline transdermal system (STS) for HIV-associated cognitive impairment: open-label report of ACTG 5090. *HIV Clin Trials.* 2007;8:437–446.

102. Kidd PM. A review of nutrients and botanicals in the integrative management of cognitive dysfunction. *Altern Med Rev.* 1999;4:144–161.

103. Jorissen BL, Brouns F, van Boxtel MP, et al. The influence of soy-derived phosphatidylserine on cognition in age-associated memory impairment. *Nutr Neurosci.* 2001;4:121–134.

104. Cocito L, Bianchetti A, Bossi L, Giberti L, Loeb C. GABA and phosphatidylserine in human photosensitivity: a pilot study. *Epilepsy Res.* 1994;17:49–53.

105. Thal LJ, Carta A, Clarke WR , RC, et al. A 1-year multicenter placebo-controlled study of acetyl-L-carnitine in patients with Alzheimer's disease. *Neurology.* 1996;47:705–711.

106. Brooks JO III, Yesavage JA, Carta A, Bravi D. Acetyl-L-carnitine slows decline in younger patients with Alzheimer's disease: a reanalysis of a double-blind, placebo-controlled study using the trilinear approach. *Int Psychogeriatr.* 1998;10:193–203.

107. Bonavita E. Study of the efficacy and tolerability of L-acetylcarnitine therapy in the senile brain. *Int J Clin Pharmacol Ther Toxicol.* 1986;24:511–516.

108. Fariello RG, Zeeman E, Golden GT, Reyes PT, Ramacci T. Transient seizure activity induced by acetylcarnitine. *Neuropharmacology.* 1984;23:585–587.

109. Badmaev V. *Bacopin (Bacopa Monniera): A Memory Enhancer From Ayurveda.* Piscataway, NJ: Sabinsa Corporation; 1998.

110. Singh RH, Singh L. Studies on the anti-anxiety effect of the medyha rasayana drug, Brahmi (*Bacopa monniera* Wettest)—part 1. *J Res Ayur Siddha.* 1980;1:133–148.

111. Calabrese C, Gregory WL, Leo M, Kraemer D, Bone K, Oken B. Effects of a standardized *Bacopa monnieri* extract on cognitive performance, anxiety, and depression in the elderly: a randomized, double-blind, placebo-controlled trial. *J Altern Complement Med.* 2008;14:707–713.

112. Khan R, Krishnakumar A, Paulose CS. Decreased glutamate receptor binding and NMDA R1 gene expression in hippocampus of pilocarpine-induced epileptic rats: neuroprotective role of *Bacopa monnieri* extract. *Epilepsy Behav.* 2008;12:54–60.

113. Otomo E, Atarashi J, Araki G, et al. Comparison of vinpocetine with ifenprodil tartrate and dihydroergotoxine mesylate treatment and results of long-term treatment with vinpocetine. *Curr Therapeutic Res.* 1985;37:811–821.

114. Tamaki N, Kusunoki T, Matsumoto S. The effect of vinpocetine on cerebral blood flow in patients with cerebrovascular disorders. *Ther Hung.* 1985;33:13–21.

115. Kuzuya F. Effects of vinpocetine on platelet aggregability and erythrocyte deformability. *Ther Hung.* 1985;33:22–34.

116. Balestreri R, Fontana L, Astengo F. A double-blind placebo controlled evaluation of the safety and efficacy of vinpocetine in the treatment of patients with chronic vascular senile cerebral dysfunction. *J Am Geriatr Soc.* 1987;35:425–430.

117. Hindmarch I, Fuchs H, Erzigkeit H. Efficacy and tolerance of vinpocetine in ambulant patients suffering from mild to moderate organic psychosyndromes. *Int Clin Psychopharmacol.* 1991;6:31–43.

118. Thal LJ, Salmon DP, Lasker B, Bower D, Klauber MR. The safety and lack of efficacy of vinpocetine in Alzheimer's disease. *J Am Geriatr Soc.* 1989;37:515–520.

119. Vohora D, Saraogi P, Yazdani MA, Bhowmik M, Khanam R, Pillai KK. Recent advances in adjunctive therapy for epilepsy: focus on sodium channel blockers as third-generation antiepileptic drugs. *Drugs Today.* 2010;46:265–277.

120. Struder HK, Hollmann W, Platen P, Donike M, Gotzmann A, Weber K. Influence of paroxetine, branched-chain amino acids and tyrosine on neuroendocrine system responses and fatigue in humans. *Horm Metab Res.* 1998;30:188–194.

121. Chinevere TD, Sawyer RD, Creer AR, Conlee RK, Parcell AC. Effects of L-tyrosine and carbohydrate ingestion on endurance exercise performance. *J Appl Physiol.* 2002;93: 1590–1597.
122. Thomas JR, Lockwood PA, Singh A, Deuster PA. Tyrosine improves working memory in a multitasking environment. *Pharmacol Biochem Behav.* 1999;64:495–500.
123. Mahoney CR, Castellani J, Kramer FM, Young A, Lieberman HR. Tyrosine supplementation mitigates working memory decrements during cold exposure. *Physiol Behav.* 2007;92:575–578.
124. Aisen PS, Schneider LS, Sano M, et al. High dose vitamin B supplementation and cognitive decline in Alzheimer's disease: a randomized controlled study. *JAMA.* 2008;300: 1774–1783.
125. Jia X, Craig LC, Aucott LS, Milne AC, McNeill G. Repeatability and validity of a food frequency questionnaire in free-living older people in relation to cognitive function. *J Nutr Health Aging.* 2008;12:735–741.
126. Plecko B, Stockler S. Vitamin B_6 dependent seizures. *Can J Neurol Sci.* 2009;36:S73–S77.
127. Mathiowetz V, Matuska KM, Murphy ME. Efficacy of an energy conservation course for persons with multiple sclerosis. *Arch Phys Med Rehabil.* 2001;82:449–456.
128. www.ampakines.org/nootropics.htm
129. Sahakian B, Morein-Zamir S. Professor's little helper. *Nature.* 2007;450:1157–1159.
130. Kaiser PR, Valko PO, Werth E, et al. Modafinil ameliorates excessive daytime sleepiness after traumatic brain injury. *Neurology.* 2010;75:1780–1785.
131. Greely H, Sahakian B, Harris J, et al. Towards responsible use of cognitive-enhancing drugs by the healthy. *Nature.* 2008;456:702–705.
132. Veena SR, Krishnaveni GV, Srinivasan K, et al. Higher maternal plasma folate but not vitamin B-12 concentrations during pregnancy are associated with better cognitive function scores in 9- to 10- year-old children in South India. *J Nutr.* 2010;140:1014–1022.
133. Monti JM, Jantos H. The roles of dopamine and serotonin, and of their receptors, in regulating sleep and waking. *Prog Brain Res.* 2008;172:625–646.
134. Wu WC, Walaas SI, Nairn AC, Greengard P. Calcium/phospholipid regulates phosphorylation of a Mr "87k" substrate protein in brain synaptosomes. *Proc Natl Acad Sci USA.* 1982;79:5249–5253.
135. Kolotushkina EV, Moldavan MG, Voronin KY, Skibo GG. The influence of *Hericium erinaceus* extract on myelination process in vitro. *Fiziol Zh.* 2003;49:38–45.
136. Mori K, Obara Y, Hirota M, et al. Nerve growth factor-inducing activity of *Hericium erinaceus* in 1321N1 human astrocytoma cells. *Biol Pharm Bull.* 2008;31:1727–1732.
137. Mori K, Inatomi S, Ouchi K, Azumi Y, Tuchida T. Improving effects of the mushroom yamabushitake (*Hericium erinaceus*) on mild cognitive impairment: a double-blind placebo-controlled clinical trial. *Phytother Res.* 2009;23:367–372.
138. Mischoulon D, Fava M. Role of S-adenosyl-L-methionine in the treatment of depression: a review of the evidence. *Am J Clin Nutr.* 2002;76:1158S–1161S.
139. Singh HK, Dhawan BN. Neuropsychopharmacological effects of the Ayurvedic nootropic *Bacopa monniera* Linn. *Indian J Pharmacol.* 1997;29:359–365.
140. Joshi H, Parle M. Brahmi rasayana improves learning and memory in mice. *Evid Based Complement Alternat Med.* 2006;3:79–85.
141. Britton A, Singh-Manoux A, Marmot M. Alcohol consumption and cognitive function in the Whitehall II Study. *Am J Epidemiol.* 2004;160:240–247.
142. Launer LJ, Feskens EJ, Kalmijn S, Kromhout D. Smoking, drinking, and thinking. The Zutphen Elderly Study. *Am J Epidemiol.* 1996;143:219–227.
143. Galanis DJ, Joseph C, Masaki KH, Petrovitch H, Ross GW, White L. A longitudinal study of drinking and cognitive performance in elderly Japanese American men: the Honolulu-Asia Aging Study. *Am J Public Health.* 2000;90:1254–1259.

144. Dufouil C, Ducimetiere P, Alperovitch A. Sex differences in the association between alcohol consumption and cognitive performance. EVA Study Group. Epidemiology of Vascular Aging. *Am J Epidemiol.* 1997;146:405–412.
145. Rodgers B, Windsor TD, Anstey KJ, Dear KB, F Jorm A, Christensen H. Non-linear relationships between cognitive function and alcohol consumption in young, middle-aged and older adults: the PATH Through Life Project. *Addiction.* 2005;100:1280–1290.

11

Managing Anxiety and Depression

Many people with epilepsy (PWE) experience symptoms of a mood disorder over their lifetimes. As many as 10% to 60% of PWE have anxiety or depression at some time, depending on how the study was done and the severity of the epilepsy. In a large Canadian study, 17% of PWE had major depression at some point in their lives as compared with 10% of people without epilepsy; 23% had some anxiety disorder, which was more than twice the rate in people without epilepsy; and nearly 1 in 3 PWE had both anxiety and depression at some time, compared with 20% of people without epilepsy (1).

Studies at comprehensive epilepsy centers, which generally care for PWE whose seizures are not controlled by antiepileptic drugs (AEDs), show a greater impact of anxiety and depression. One study found that nearly 1 in 7 patients going to an epilepsy center experienced major depression, and more than half also had symptoms of an anxiety disorder (2).

Many scientists have studied the relationships among epilepsy, anxiety, and depression and have put forward multiple explanatory theories. Notably, PWE are at much greater risk of developing anxiety and depression than people without epilepsy, *and* persons with depression are at increased risk for developing epilepsy (3). These studies suggest that there are reciprocal vulnerabilities and, likely, shared genetic and environmental risks for epilepsy and psychiatric disorders. Similar findings have also emerged for migraine and epilepsy (4).

TYPES OF ANXIETY AND DEPRESSION IN PWEs

There are different types of anxiety disorders in the general population. The most common types in PWE are phobias, generalized anxiety disorder, and panic disorder (1).

All 4 main types of depression identified in people without epilepsy also occur in PWE: major depressive disorders, dysthymic disorder, minor depression, and depressive disorder not otherwise specified. The differences between these types of depression relate to how long the symptoms last, how often they reoccur, and how severe they are. For example, major depressive disorder is defined as a recurring episode of depression involving many symptoms of depression and lasting for more than 2 weeks.

The symptoms of depression in PWE may be somewhat different than in people without epilepsy and may therefore not meet the diagnostic criteria established by psychiatrists for depression in people without epilepsy. This is a caveat for all behavioral disorders in epilepsy. In one study, nearly 3 of 4 PWE with symptoms of depression severe enough to require medical therapy did not meet these diagnostic criteria (5). Some researchers diagnose these PWE with "interictal dysphoric disorder," characterized by intermittent symptoms of irritability or frustration intermixed with feelings of great happiness, elation, or well-being as well as fear, anxiousness, low energy, bodily pains, and trouble sleeping (6–7).

People with epilepsy may have fluctuating symptoms of anxiety and depression depending on whether the person is actually having a seizure (ictal), is recovering from a very recent seizure (postictal), or has not had a seizure for some time (interictal). We focus on interictal anxiety and depression in this chapter, beginning with an overview of medical therapy and then various nonpharmacologic, complementary approaches that many PWE may try for anxiety- or depression-related symptoms, particularly before they are diagnosed with these conditions by physicians, or when physicians conclude that the symptoms are not severe enough to warrant medical therapies. Ictal depression is uncommon and often transient. Postictal depression is more common and causes greater disability but does usually resolve within hours or days without treatment. Ictal anxiety and fear are common with temporal lobe seizures but can also occur with frontal lobe seizures. Seizure control is the most effective strategy to reduce ictal anxiety. Postictal anxiety is more common than patients report or physicians recognize but, like depression, often resolves spontaneously (8). If moderate or severe, a benzodiazepine such as clonazepam can be used to treat this. Interictal affective symptoms are the most enduring and disabling affective symptoms in PWE.

OVERVIEW OF MEDICAL THERAPY FOR ANXIETY AND DEPRESSION

Anxiety disorders and depression are serious medical illnesses that should be evaluated by physicians with the appropriate training and background to recommend therapy (when medically necessary) and monitor the response to therapy. Failure to treat depression or anxiety in a PWE can significantly impair quality of life and exacerbate seizures, directly or indirectly (e.g., insomnia); lack of effective treatment may be life threatening for persons who become suicidal. Therefore, before PWE consider complementary approaches to treat anxiety or depression, they should seek appropriate medical care. If any of the following are present, the patient should be urgently evaluated by a psychiatrist: persistent symptoms of an anxiety disorder or depression despite treatment with a selective serotonin reuptake inhibitor (SSRI) and a selective norepinephrine reuptake inhibitor (SNRI); symptoms of depression together with thoughts of suicide (suicidal ideation) or indications of psychosis (distorted or incoherent sense of objective reality in the external world, often with delusions or hallucinations); a history of previous depression that did not respond to medical therapies; or a history of bipolar disorder (sometimes called *manic-depressive* disorder). Also, patients with suicidal thoughts should be asked if they have a plan to carry out the suicide. If so, it should be considered an emergency until they are evaluated by a psychiatrist.

A PWE can have anxiety and depression at the same time. This is important because the choices of available medical and complementary therapies are different from if only anxiety or depression is present.

Before treatment is started, the physician should be sure that anxiety or depression in a particular patient is not related to one or more AEDs that the patient is taking or has recently stopped taking. The side effects of some AEDs such as phenobarbital, levetiracetam, zonisamide, topiramate, and tiagabine may be mistaken for an anxiety disorder or depression. On the other hand, some AEDs can reduce or eliminate symptoms of an underlying anxiety disorder or depression, such as valproate, lamotrigine, gabapentin, and pregabalin. This may lead to the emergence of anxiety- or depression-related symptoms associated with the underlying conditions if these AEDs are stopped. The clinical challenge is to identify temporal relations between introduction (or increased dose, decreased dose, or cessation) of an AED and behavioral symptoms. Although some AEDs (e.g., levetiracetam) are well known to cause behavioral side effects, other AEDs (e.g., lamotrigine, gabapentin) that often improve behavior can cause psychiatric symptoms in some patients (9–10). Further, a temporal relationship does not establish causation. Clinically, one must remain open-minded about a possible relation of an AED and either a negative or positive behavioral change but also avoid jumping to a conclusion. Systematic observation and humility are essential.

MEDICAL THERAPIES FOR ANXIETY AND DEPRESSION IN PWE

Persons diagnosed with anxiety disorders or depression that significantly interferes with quality of life are usually started on drug therapy that targets neurotransmitters that influence anxiety and depression, including serotonin and norepinephrine (11). An SSRI is usually started first, especially one that treats anxiety disorders and depression since they so often occur together. If an SSRI does not work after a sufficiently long period (at least several weeks) or if side effects are bothersome, then the physician may prescribe a drug that works as a selective serotonin and norepinephrine reuptake inhibitor (SNRI).

Drugs classified as benzodiazepines (including alprazolam, clonazepam, diazepam, and lorazepam) may be recommended for anxiety disorders for short periods and occasionally are taken with antidepressants. Benzodiazepines pose a 2-edged sword for PWE. These drugs are very effective for reducing seizures for limited periods. Then, as tolerance develops, they are less effective for controlling seizures or reducing anxiety. However, for those who are treated for more than 1 to 2 weeks on these drugs, reduction or discontinuation of the drugs can lead to a significant increase in anxiety and/or seizure activity. Therefore, after several weeks of use, if the goal is to reduce or eliminate these drugs, they should be tapered gradually. Another medication used for generalized anxiety disorder is buspirone, which (unlike benzodiazepines) does not potentially cause tolerance, addiction, or problems when it is stopped.

Medical treatment of anxiety disorders and depression for PWE is generally similar to that for people without epilepsy. Unfortunately, there are very few studies on the effectiveness and safety of these medications in PWE. Physicians should check for possible interactions between the AEDs taken by PWE and the new medication(s) prescribed for the mood disorder and make dosage adjustments accordingly. In addition, drugs should be avoided that may exacerbate side effects that are already occurring from AEDs (such as trouble falling asleep).

Physicians may hesitate to start an SSRI or SNRI in PWE because of concerns that seizures may increase in frequency or severity. While this has not been extensively evaluated by clinical research, at least one study in 97 PWE with depression suggested that the SSRI sertraline does not significantly worsen seizures (5). Other studies support that antidepressant and other psychiatric drugs are safe for the large majority of PWE (12).

As mentioned, certain AEDs may improve symptoms of anxiety and depression (11), and some physicians might accordingly adjust the AEDs that a PWE is taking in an effort to treat both the seizures and the mood disorder, especially when seizure control is good and anxiety- or depression-related symptoms are mild.

COMPLEMENTARY APPROACHES FOR THE MANAGEMENT OF ANXIETY AND DEPRESSION

Few research studies have evaluated the safety and effectiveness of complementary treatments for the treatment of anxiety and depression in PWE. While there are more such studies in people without epilepsy who have anxiety or depression, there are not enough studies in most instances to clearly determine the benefits or risks of these treatments, whether in PWE or not.

NEUROBEHAVIORAL APPROACHES

Neurobehavioral approaches are a subset of the category of complementary and alternative medical (CAM) therapies as described by the National Center for Complementary and Alternative Medicine, called mind-body medicine (13). They are designed to induce relaxation and enhance the mind's capacity to affect bodily function and modulate the body and mind's response to stress (14). Mind-body medicine is the most commonly used form of CAM by adults with chronic neurologic conditions, and the specific techniques most commonly used by those with neurologic conditions were deep breathing exercises, meditation, and yoga (19%, 13%, and 7%, respectively) (15–16).

The use of cognitive behavioral therapy (CBT) and a related method, acceptance and commitment therapy, for control of seizures is discussed in Chapter 6 (Neurobehavioral Approaches). These techniques can be effective in treating anxiety disorders and depression, including in PWE (17–19). Other psychologically based therapies and mind–body techniques were used in PWE with evidence of reduced seizure activity and improved mood (20); these methods include induction of relaxation through yoga and meditation (21–22). These studies do not definitively prove a benefit for PWE in seizures or mood. However, 2 of 3 trials found that CBT reduced depression among PWE, one trial found combined relaxation and behavior modification reduced anxiety, and some studies found that yoga and relaxation techniques reduced depressive symptoms (23–26).

One promising study compared CBT with usual counseling in adolescents who were recently diagnosed with epilepsy to see if depression could be prevented in those at risk (27). Cognitive behavioral therapy and counseling were provided weekly for 2 months and then monthly for 4 months. Symptoms of depressive disorders improved significantly in the patients treated with CBT as compared with those who received counseling.

A home-based treatment for depression in adults with epilepsy using a form of CBT called mindfulness-based CBT was delivered by the Internet or telephone and described in a recently published study (28). The intervention consisted of eight 1-hour sessions with discussions, instruction, and skill-building activities addressing depression, epilepsy, and the role of mindfulness and cognitive behavior change. The Internet aspect of the intervention allowed for discussions, viewing session materials, and posting between sessions on a secure Web site. The findings in the research participants who received the intervention were compared with those who were put on a waiting list. The intervention groups showed a significant decline in depressive symptoms over the wait-list group, and the improvement persisted for over 8 weeks.

BIOLOGICALLY BASED PRACTICES

Biologically based practices are another subset of CAM therapies and include the use of substances found in nature such as herbs, foods, vitamins, and animal compounds. This group of practices was the most commonly used form of CAM by the U.S. general population in 2007 (29).

The use of herb-derived products by PWE is discussed in Chapter 2 (Herbal Remedies). An analysis of publications on use of herbal remedies by PWE found that St. John's wort is very commonly (13%) taken (30). Kava is also frequently taken by PWE (31). These findings suggest that some PWE use herbal remedies to treat anxiety and depression. While no research has specifically studied the efficacy of herbal medicines for anxiety or depression in PWE, published studies suggest benefit of St. John's wort in treating mild to moderate depression and kava for generalized anxiety (12, 32–34). Other herbal remedies anecdotally reported to improve anxiety or depression include passionflower extracts and rosenroot (35–36). There is insufficient evidence about other herbal remedies alone or in combination with antidepressants, mood stabilizers, or benzodiazepines (37–38).

Other natural products that may improve symptoms of anxiety or depression include ω-3 fatty acids, which is the most commonly taken biologically based product by U.S. Americans in a 2007 survey; S-adenosylmethionine (SAM-e); and combinations of L-lysine, L-arginine, and magnesium-containing dietary supplements (12, 29, 35, 39).

People with epilepsy who try one or more of these natural products should inform their physician, since these products, especially SAM-e and St. John's wort, could affect the blood levels of other medications, including AEDs. In addition, they may cause side effects that the physician might otherwise attribute to an AED. St. John's wort, for example, may cause overstimulation; kava can bring on headache and gastrointestinal complaints as well as adversely affect liver function; and SAM-e may decrease appetite and cause dry mouth, nervousness, and trouble falling asleep (32).

ENERGY MEDICINE

This category of CAM includes therapeutic touch, Reiki, and acupuncture. No studies specifically assess the effect of these techniques on PWE with anxiety or depression. Studies of acupuncture in people without epilepsy fail to show a consistent beneficial effect for anxiety or depression compared with a waitlist control or sham acupuncture control (40). One comprehensive review of published clinical research did find a benefit of acupuncture for depression that developed after a stroke (41).

EXERCISE

Physical exercise can reduce anxiety and depression in the general population (42–43). In PWE, physical exercise is associated with significantly lower levels of depression, and improved mood can occur within 4 weeks of an exercise program (44). High-energy exercise and frequent aerobic exercise (at least 3 to 5 times per week) appear to reduce symptoms of depression more than less frequent or lower-energy exercise (45).

CONCLUSION

Many complementary approaches to treat anxiety and depression have been studied, most often in PWE. Convincing evidence for the effectiveness of these approaches is not presently available, largely owing to the challenges in designing definitive research studies using these treatments. However, there is general agreement that neurobehavioral approaches are safe. Additional research will hopefully further clarify whether any of these treatments work for PWE and, if they do, who is most likely to benefit.

People with epilepsy should be active partners in managing their health. It is a 2-way street: patients need to share information about all their medical and CAM therapies, and physician need to maintain an open mind to therapies that have not been fully evaluated. A key to a successful physician-patient partnership is full and open discussion of the pros and cons of all possible treatments, including those that PWEs have access to over the counter or through other health care providers (such as acupuncture) and that they are considering trying, so that fully informed choices are made.

REFERENCES

1. Tellez-Zenteno JF, Pattern SB, Jette N, Williams J, Wiebe S. Psychiatric comorbidity in epilepsy: a population-based analysis. *Epilepsia.* 2007;48:2336–2344.
2. Kanner AM, Barry JJ, Gilliam F, Hermann B, Meador KJ. Anxiety disorders, sub-syndromic depressive episodes and major depressive episodes: do they differ on their impact on the quality of life of patients with epilepsy? *Epilepsia.* 2010;51:1152–1158.
3. Hesdorffer DC, Hauser WA, Ludvigsson P, Olafsson E, Kjartansson O. Depression and attempted suicide as risk factors for incident unprovoked seizures and epilepsy. *Ann Neurol.* 2006;59:35–41.
4. Tikka-Kleemola P, Artto V, Vepsalainen S, et al. A visual migraine aura locus maps to 9q21-q22. *Neurology.* 2010;74:1171–1177.
5. Kanner AM, Kozak AM, Frey M. The use of sertraline in patients with epilepsy: is it safe? *Epilepsy Behav.* 2000;1:100–105.
6. Blumer D, Altshuler LL. Affective disorders. In: Engel J, Pedley TA, eds. *Epilepsy: A Comprehensive Textbook.* Vol. 2. Philadelphia, PA: Lippincott-Raven; 1998:2083–2099.
7. Mula M, Jauch R, Cavanna A, et al. Clinical and psychopathological definition of the interictal dysphoric disorder of epilepsy. *Epilepsia.* 2008;49:650–656.
8. Kanner AM, Trimble M, Schmitz B. Postictal affective episodes. *Epilepsy Behav.* 2010;19:156–158.
9. Ettinger AB, Weisbrot DM, Saracco J, Dhoon A, Kanner A, Devinsky O. Positive and negative psychotropic effects of lamotrigine in patients with epilepsy and mental retardation. *Epilepsia.* 1998;39:874–877.
10. Wolf SM, Shinnar S, Kang H, Gil KB, Moshe SL. Gabapentin toxicity in children manifesting as behavioral changes. *Epilepsia.* 1995;36:1203–1205.
11. Huffman JC, Alpert JE. An approach to the psychopharmacologic care of patients: antidepressants, antipsychotics, anxiolytics, mood stabilizers, and natural remedies. *Med Clin N Am.* 2010;94:1141–1160.
12. Gross A, Devinsky O, Westbrook LE, Wharton AH, Alper K. Psychotropic medication use in patients with epilepsy: effect on seizure frequency. *J Neuropsychiatry Clin Neurosci.* 2000;12:458–464.
13. What is complementary and alternative medicine? National Center for Complementary and Alternative Medicine Web site. http://nccam.nih.gov/health/whatiscam/. Accessed April 18, 2012.

14. Dusek JA, Benon H. Mind-body medicine: a model of the comparative clinical impact of the acute stress and relaxation responses. *Minn Med.* 2009;92:47–50.
15. Wells RE, Phillips RS, Schachter SC, McCarty EP. Complementary and alternative medicine use among U.S. adults with common neurological conditions. *J Neurol.* 2010;257: 1822–1831.
16. Wells RE, Phillips RS, McCarty EP. Patterns of mind-body therapies in adults with common neurological conditions. *Neuroepidemiology.* 2011;36:46–51.
17. Dahl JC, Lundgren TL. Conditioning mechanisms, behavioral technology, and contextual behavior therapy. In: Schachter SC, Holmes GL, Trenite DGAK, eds. *Behavioral Aspects of Epilepsy: Principles & Practice.* New York, NY: Demos Medical Publishing; 2008: 245–252.
18. Gilliam FG, Black KJ, Carter J, et al. Depression and health outcomes in epilepsy: a randomized trial. Presented at the 61st Annual Meeting of the American Academy of Neurology; April 25–May 2, 2009; Seattle, WA.
19. Linden M, Zubraegel D, Baer T, Franke U, Schlattmann P. Efficacy of cognitive behaviour therapy in generalized anxiety disorders. Results of a controlled clinical trial (Berlin CBT-GAD Study). *Psychother Psychosom.* 2005;74:36–42.
20. Mittan R. Psychosocial treatment programs in epilepsy: a review. *Epilepsy Behav.* 2009;16:371–380.
21. Lansky EP, St Louis EK. Transcendental meditation: a double-edged sword in epilepsy? *Epilepsy Behav.* 2006;9:394–400.
22. Yardi N. Yoga for control of epilepsy. *Seizure.* 2001;10:7–12.
23. Jorm AF, Morgan AJ, Hetrick SE. Relaxation for depression. *Cochrane Database Syst Rev.* 2008;4:CD007142.
24. Pilkington K, Kirkwood G, Rampes H, Richardson J. Yoga for depression: The research evidence. *J Affect Disord.* 2005;89:13–24.
25. Ramaratnam S, Sridharan K. Yoga for epilepsy. *Cochrane Database Syst Rev.* 2000;3: CD001524.
26. Ramaratnam S, Baker G, Goldstein L. Psychological treatments for epilepsy. *Cochrane Database Syst Rev.* 2008;3:CD002029.
27. Martinovic Z, Simonovic P, Djokic R. Preventing depression in adolescents with epilepsy. *Epilepsy Behav.* 2006;9:619–624.
28. Walker ER, Obolensky N, Dini S, Thompson NJ. Formative and process evaluations of a cognitive-behavioral therapy and mindfulness intervention for people with epilepsy and depression. *Epilepsy Behav.* 2010;19:239–246.
29. Barnes PM, Bloom B, Nahin RL. Complementary and alternative medicine use among adults and children: United States, 2007. *Natl Health Stat Rep.* 2008;10:1–23.
30. Ekstein D, Schachter SC. Natural products in epilepsy—the present situation and perspectives for the future. *Pharmaceuticals.* 2010;3:1426–1445.
31. Sirven JI, Drazkowski JF, Zimmerman RS, Bortz JJ, Shulman DL, Macleish M. Complementary/alternative medicine for epilepsy in Arizona. *Neurology.* 2003;61:576–577.
32. Larzelere MM, Campbell JS, Robertson M. Complementary and alternative medicine usage for behavioral health indications. *Prim Care Clin Office Pract.* 2010;37:213–236.
33. Sarris J, Kavanagh DJ. Kava and St. John's wort: current evidence for use in mood and anxiety disorders. *J Altern Complement Med.* 2009;15:827–836.
34. Sarris J, LaPorte E, Schweitzer I. Kava: a comprehensive review of efficacy, safety, and psychopharmacology. *Aust N Z J Psychiatry.* 2011;45:27–35.
35. Lakhan SE, Vieira KF. Nutritional and herbal supplements for anxiety and anxiety-related disorders: systematic review. *Nutr J.* 2010;9:42–56.
36. Panossian A, Wikman G, Sarris J. Rosenroot (*Rhodiola rosea*): traditional use, chemical composition, pharmacology and clinical efficacy. *Phytomedicine.* 2010;17:481–493.

37. Sarris J. Herbal medicines in the treatment of psychiatric disorders: a systematic review. *Phytother Res*. 2007;21:703–716.
38. Sarris J, Kavanagh DJ, Byrne G. Adjuvant use of nutritional and herbal medicines with antidepressants, mood stabilizers and benzodiazepines. *J Psychiatr Res*. 2010;44:32–41.
39. Kraguljac NV, Montori VM, Pavuluri M, Chai HS, Wilson BS, Unal SS. Efficacy of omega-3 fatty acids in mood disorders—a systematic review and metaanalysis. *Psychopharmacol Bull*. 2009;42:39–54.
40. Pilkington K. Anxiety, depression and acupuncture: a review of the clinical research. *Auton Neurosci*. 2010;157:91–95.
41. Smith CA, Hay PP, Macpherson H. Acupuncture for depression. *Cochrane Database Syst Rev*. 2010;1:CD004046.
42. Greist JH, Klein MH, Eischens RR, Faris J, Furman AS, Morgan WP. Running for treatment of depression. *Comp Psychiatry*. 1979;20:41–54.
43. Putruzzello SJ, Landers DM, Hatfield BD, Kubitz KA, Salazar W. A meta-analysis on the anxiety-reducing effects of acute and chronic exercise. *Sports Med*. 1991;11:143–182.
44. Arida RM, Scorza FA, da Silva SG, Schachter SC, Cavalheiro EA. The potential role of physical exercise in the treatment of epilepsy. *Epilepsy Behav*. 2010;17:432–435.
45. Saeed SA, Antonacci DJ, Bloch RM. Exercise, yoga, and meditation for depressive and anxiety disorders. *Am Fam Physician*; 2010;81:981–986.

12

Epilepsy and Stress

STRESS AND THE BODY

The word *stress* derives from *distress*. Stress refers to any physical or emotional challenge that leads to bodily or psychological tension. In this chapter, stress refers to emotional or psychosocial stress. To understand the effects of stress on the human brain and its role in people with epilepsy (PWE), it is important to recognize its effects on the body. The body's innate and reflexive ability to handle stress is a necessity for survival. The fight or flight response enables us to perform with maximal alertness and ability under dangerous or threatening conditions. The American physiologist Walter Bradford Cannon first described this phenomenon in the early 20th century after discovering that animals respond to threat with intense activation of the sympathetic nervous system.

Acute stress responses activate the sympathetic nervous system and, through it, the adrenal medulla to release norepinephrine and epinephrine; they also activate the hypothalamic-pituitary-adrenocortical axis that releases the glucocorticoid steroid hormone cortisol (1). This biological response initiated in the brain's limbic system is in full force within seconds of a perceived threat. Widespread and profound effects occur throughout the body. The heart rate is accelerated, with a resultant increase in cardiac output. Blood is shunted away from the skin and gastrointestinal tract to vital organs and skeletal muscle. Respiration becomes rapid, blood pressure and blood sugar elevate, pain perception decreases, and pupils dilate.

These bodily effects help to flee or fight an attacker, but this response is often initiated by minor stressors of everyday life: being late for meetings, relationship difficulty, traffic jams, financial issues, and public speaking engagements may trigger intense physiological responses originally designed for readying our bodies for the fight of our life. The seemingly ubiquitous overactivity of the stress response in our society may reflect a variety of factors: overstimulation, excess work, stimulants (e.g., caffeine), poor dietary habits (e.g., excess carbohydrates), poor sleep habits (e.g., insomnia), lack of physical activity, and others. Regardless

167

of the cause, people who spend much of their lives in a hypervigilant state may experience physical consequences.

Stress may contribute to diseases in all organ systems. However, while many medical illnesses can be exacerbated or caused by emotional stress, the exact incidence of stress-related illness or the magnitude of stress as a factor in certain disorders, like cancer, is unknown. Quantifying the effects of chronic stress relative to other risk factors for a given disease in any individual is difficult. People differ substantially in their physical and psychological responses to the same emotional stress. Genetic and environmentally derived character and personality traits determine our personal stress response to potential threats. Further, individuals who respond intensely to physical stresses, like vigorous exercise, may also respond intensely to psychological stress.

Singh and colleagues (2) separated healthy men into 2 groups based on the magnitude of their stress-induced adrenocorticotropic hormone (ACTH) response, measured in the blood after intense physical exercise. Those individuals who were classified as high responders based on increased ACTH levels during strenuous exercise also had elevated ACTH in response to the psychological stress of performing calculations and to an intense interview process.

Stress is often cited as an etiologic factor in heart disease. Activation of the sympathetic nervous system can accelerate the development of atherosclerosis, hypertension, and even insulin resistance (3). While still controversial as a cause of essential hypertension, chronic exposure to high stress can elevate blood pressure over sustained periods (4). Moreover, stress reduction through techniques like transcendental meditation can help control hypertension (5).

Stress can contribute to unhealthy behaviors including smoking, sedentary lifestyle, and obesity, all of which can contribute to atherosclerosis, thereby increasing the risk for heart attack and stroke (6). Personality type correlates with risk of heart disease (7). Some researchers believe that individuals who exhibit Type A behavior, defined as a pattern of anger, aggravation, irritability, impatience, or time urgency, may have twice the risk for heart disease compared with those who do not. Other studies confirm the role of depression, anxiety, hostility, and trait anger as risk factors for coronary heart disease, while others challenge this association (8–9). Type A behaviors as a response to stress correlate with risk factors for coronary artery disease, including elevated blood pressure and increased platelet activation (10–11).

The immune system is adversely affected by chronic stress. A systematic review of all prospective studies showed a significant correlation between recurrence of herpes simplex virus (HSV) infection and psychosocial stress (12). This effect was greater for psychosocial than for physical stresses and stronger for HSV1 or labial infections. This suggests that stress can impair the function of T lymphocytes, which combat viral infections. The immune system ages more rapidly under stress, increasing susceptibility to infections (13). Stress-induced aging and impairment of T lymphocytes' (CD8 or cytotoxic cells) functions render them less capable of fighting off infections like cytomegalovirus, HSV, and HIV. Stress also impairs the immune function of caregivers whose family members have dementia. When compared with noncaregiving older adults, caregivers demonstrate poorer responses to vaccines, impaired control of latent viruses, exaggerated production of inflammatory mediators, and accelerated cellular aging (14).

Stress-induced impairment of immune function via T-cell senescence was suggested as a factor in the initiation of various cancers (13). While the effects of psychosocial stress as an initial cause of cancer remains controversial, there is less controversy about the increased likelihood of cancer progression and a diminished response to cancer treatments in those who experience high levels of emotional distress (15). Many cancer centers use stress reduction and stress management programs using techniques from yoga to mindfulness training. While quality-of-life benefits occur in cancer patients who participate in stress management programs, conclusive data on improved treatment outcomes are still lacking (16).

STRESS AND THE BRAIN

The protean effects of stress on the body may adversely affect the brain. Coronary artery disease may result in myocardial infarction, which can lead to clot formation in the heart's left atrium or ventricle. This can cause embolic stroke and brain injury. Similarly, prolonged hypertension can accelerate atherosclerosis, narrow blood vessel lumens, and reduce delivery of oxygen and nutrients to the brain as well as increase the risk of stroke. Lung, breast or other cancers that grow more rapidly under the influence of emotional stress may spread to the brain. Reduced immunity increases the risk of neurologic infections with herpes virus and HIV. Any of these brain disorders can cause seizures and epilepsy.

Stress can directly impair brain function in addition to its indirect effects via the heart, blood vessels, and immune system. Research on how stress affects brain function focuses on attention and memory. To acquire and retain information, one must attend to the material that is presented or experienced. Working memory, the ability to actively hold information in the mind for use in cognition, is performed by the prefrontal cortex (PFC). Attention and working memory can be assessed by verbally or visually presenting a series of digits to subjects and then asking them to repeat the numbers back. In a study on this cognitive task in 40 men under normal and emotionally stressful conditions, the men responded more slowly and less accurately while under stress (17). Elevated salivary cortisol levels confirmed a physical effect of a stressful simulated job interview procedure on the men.

The effects of psychosocial stress on the frontal lobe are reversible (18). Functional magnetic resonance imaging (MRI) of the brain was used to assess PFC activity and its functional connections with the parietal lobe following prolonged stressful and nonstressful periods. The 20 healthy volunteers had abnormal functional MRI responses to an attention-shifting task performed after 1 month of increased psychosocial stress. The degree of self-reported stress was confirmed using a validated stress rating scale, the Cohen perceived stress scale. The healthy subjects' functional MRIs normalized after a 1-month period of reduced stress. While the effects of stress on the brain in these subjects were reversible, it is not known whether longer periods of intense psychosocial stress can lead to permanent changes in PFC cortical network activity.

Along with working memory, stress affects another crucial memory function, declarative memory. Declarative memory refers to both episodic memory, memory for life events, and semantic memory (i.e., memory for facts). While working memory depends largely on the PFC, declarative memory depends largely on medial temporal lobe structures including the hippocampus and parahippocampal cortex. Interestingly, glucocorticoid (cortisol) receptors are present in PFC and temporal lobe memory structures, allowing them to respond to stressful situations but also rendering them vulnerable to the harmful effects of stress (19). The exact role of the corticoids, including the glucocorticoids and the mineralcorticoids (e.g., aldosterone), in the homeostatic function of memory centers is the subject of ongoing investigation. These adrenal hormones can activate mesial temporal areas, including the dentate gyrus, and may facilitate the generation of new neurons (20). Stress-related changes in the levels of these hormones, may modulate cell generation, neuronal plasticity, learning, cell vulnerability, and death.

Stress may initiate or exacerbate memory deficits in those at risk for Alzheimer disease (21–23). However, emotional stress also affects patients with brain disorders involving motor and immune systems. Patients with Parkinson disease freeze more often while walking under stressful conditions, possibly owing to effects of stress on dopaminergic activity (24–25). Multiple sclerosis (MS), an autoimmune disorder, may worsen in response to stress. Civilians with MS in Israel had more frequent disease exacerbation after exposure to the hostilities of war (26). Similarly, exacerbations in women with MS were linked to the number of stressful life experiences they experienced (27).

STRESS AND EPILEPSY

Psychosocial stress may not cause the molecular or structural brain alterations responsible for epilepsy, but it can provoke seizures in susceptible people. Studies of first seizures in adults link severe life stressors to occurrence of first seizure (28). In most adults, the stress may be the agent that provokes the development of one or more seizures either indirectly through sleep deprivation or directly. Without the psychosocial stress, these individuals might never have seizures. A Danish study examined the incidence of first diagnosis of epilepsy in parents who had lost a child younger than 18 years, finding a higher rate of epilepsy compared with parents who had not (29). Additionally, the risk of a first seizure was greatest soon after the loss. Similarly, newly recruited Israeli soldiers attached to combat units are more likely to have first seizures than young recruits working in administration or maintenance jobs (30). The difference in seizure incidence was attributed to the emotional stress of combat.

Patients commonly report that stress triggers seizures (31–33). In a survey of 210 PWE, psychological distress was the most important quality-of-life indicator and surpassed seizure frequency, medication side effects, and age of epilepsy onset (34). Because emotional stress may lead to impaired sleep or excess alcohol consumption, independent risk factors for seizures, it may be difficult to attribute a breakthrough seizure to a given stress. However, stress is still initiating the sequence of events leading up to the seizure. In at least 6 separate surveys of PWE, stress was perceived to be the most frequent factor that provokes seizures (33, 35–38). Notably, the relation between stress and increased seizures is independent of associated sleep deprivation or medication nonadherence in one study (39). A woman with epilepsy monitored on continuous video electroencephalogram had frequent absence seizures only when she was asked to speak about her history of sexual abuse, her epilepsy, or her father's illness (40). In Croatia, children who were seizure-free before the war and on stable medications for at least 1 year were studied after the onset of hostilities. Seizures were more frequent among those living in war zones than peaceful regions (41). Many children had seizures after intense emotional events (e.g., presence during a bombing, having their father leave for the army, or witnessing a parent being taken to a prison camp).

The relationship between stress and epilepsy may be 2-way. Just as stress can be a common provocative factor for seizures, seizures can induce stress responses in the brain and body. Adrenocorticotropic hormone and cortisol levels are increased after complex partial and generalized tonic-clonic seizures (42–43). In PWE, regulation of the hypothalamic-pituitary-adrenal axis may be impaired with elevated cortisol levels continuing for prolonged periods after stressful events. (43–44).

Animal studies shed light on the potential mechanisms in stress-induced seizures. In a temporal lobe model of epilepsy, stress severely impaired inhibitory GABA-ergic activity, reducing the seizure threshold in the amygdala (45). In addition, repetitive stress elevates corticosteroid levels in the temporal lobe, accelerating epileptogenesis and lowering seizure threshold in animal models (46). Finally, to cope with stress, the brain releases endogenous benzodiazepine-like compounds that prevent injury (47). Further studies are needed to determine whether this coping mechanism is functioning properly in brain regions that produce seizures.

Just as stress affects seizure control and quality of life for PWE, epilepsy is associated with unique stressors and comorbidities that may further impair coping abilities. A 2005 population-based health survey of California adults identified serious psychological distress more frequently in PWE compared with the general population (48). The survey identified higher rates of feeling nervous, hopeless, restless, depressed, or worthless in those with epilepsy. Moreover, depressed and negative feelings have been associated with worse prognosis for seizure control. In one recent study, optimistic patients had better seizure outcomes than those with persistent negative assessments of their personal health (49). Thus, while patients cite stress as the reason for their depressed feelings, depression occurs at a greater incidence in PWE, independent of stress (50–51). In many cases, the presence of depression likely accounts for the frequent feelings of distress reported by many with epilepsy (32). It is therefore critically important that PWE who voice feelings of depression be offered medical and nonmedical treatment for depression along with stress reduction measures.

REFERENCES

1. Goldstein DS. Adrenal responses to stress. *Cell Mol Neurobiol.* 2010;30:1433–1440.
2. Singh A, Petrides JS, Gold PW. Differential hypothalamic-pituitary-adrenal axis reactivity to psychological and physical stress. *J Clin Endocrinol Metab.* 1999;84:1944–1948.
3. Esler M, Kaye D. Sympathetic nervous system activation in essential hypertension, cardiac failure and psychosomatic heart disease. *J Cardiovasc Pharmacol.* 2000;35:S1–S7.
4. Sparrenberger F, Cichelero FT, Ascoli AM, et al. Does psychosocial stress cause hypertension? A systematic review of observational studies. *J Hum Hypertens.* 2009;23:12–19.
5. Rainforth MV, Schneider RH, Nidich SI, Gaylord-King C, Salerno JW, Anderson JW. Stress reduction programs in patients with elevated blood pressure: a systematic review and meta-analysis. *Curr Hypertens Rep.* 2007;9:520–528.
6. Mainous AG III, Everett CJ, Diaz VA, Player MS, Gebregziabher M, Smith DW. Life stress and atherosclerosis: a pathway through unhealthy lifestyle. *Int J Psychiatry Med.* 2010;40:147–161.
7. Kent LK, Shapiro PA. Depression and related psychological factors in heart disease. *Harv Rev Psychiatry.* 2009;17:377–388.
8. Boyle SH, Michalek JE, Suarez EC. Covariation of psychological attributes and incident coronary heart disease in U.S. Air Force veterans of the Vietnam war. *Psychosom Med.* 2006;68:844–850.
9. Shekelle RB, Hulley SB Neaton JD, et al. The MRFIT behavior pattern study. II. Type A behavior and incidence of coronary heart disease. *Am J Epidemiol.* 1985;122:559–570.
10. Brondolo E, Rieppi R, Eriskon SA, et al. Hostility, interpersonal interactions, and ambulatory blood pressure. *Psychosom Med.* 2003;65:1003–1011.
11. Markovitz J. Hostility is associated with increased platelet activation in coronary artery disease. *Psychosom Med.* 1998;60:586–591.
12. Chida Y, Mao X. Does psychosocial stress predict symptomatic herpes simplex virus recurrence? A meta-analytic investigation on prospective studies. *Brain Behav Immun.* 2009;23:917–925.
13. Effros EB. Telomere/telomerase dynamics within the human immune system: effect of chronic infection and stress. *Exp Gerontol.* 2010;46:135–140.
14. Gouin JP, Hantsoo L, Kiecolt-Glaser JK. Immune dysregulation and chronic stress among older adults: a review. *Neuroimmodulation.* 2008;15:251–259.
15. Moreno-Smith M, Lutgendorf SK, Sood AK. Impact of stress on cancer metastasis. *Future Oncol.* 2010;6:1863–1881.
16. Lutgendorf SK, Sood AK, Antoni MH. Host factors and cancer progression: biobehavioral signaling pathways and interventions. *J Clin Oncol.* 2010;28:4094–4099.
17. Schoofs D, Preuss D, Wolf OT. Psychosocial stress induces working memory impairments in an n-back paradigm. *Psychoneuroendocrinology.* 2008;33:643–653.
18. Liston C, McEwen BS, Casey BJ. Psychosocial stress reversibly disrupts prefrontal processing and attentional control. *Proc Natl Acad Sci USA.* 2009;106:912–917.
19. Weerda R, Muehlhan M, Wolf OT, Thiel CM. Effects of acute psychosocial stress on working memory related brain activity in men. *Hum Brain Mapp.* 2010;31:1418–1429.

20. Wong EY, Herbert J. Roles of mineralocorticoids and glucocorticoid receptors in the regulation of progenitor proliferation in the adult hippocampus. *Eur J Neurosci.* 2005;22: 785–792.
21. Simard M, Hudon C, van Reekum R. Psychological distress and risk for dementia. *Curr Psychiatry Rep.* 2009;11:41–47.
22. Tran TT, Srivareerat M, Alkadhi KA. Chronic psychosocial stress triggers cognitive impairment in a novel at-risk model of Alzheimer disease. *Neurobiol Dis.* 2010;37: 756–763.
23. Alkadhi KA, Srivareerat M, Tran TT. Intensification of long-term memory deficit by chronic stress and prevention by nicotine in a rat model of Alzheimer disease. *Mol Cell Neurosci.* 2010;45:289–296.
24. Rahman S, Griffin HJ, Quinn NP, Jahanshahi M. The factors that induce or overcome freezing of gait in Parkinson's disease. *Behav Neurol.* 2008;19:127–136.
25. Metz GA. Stress as a modulator of motor system function and pathology. *Rev Neurosci.* 2007;18:209–222.
26. Golan D, Somer E, Dishon S, Cuzin-Disegni L, Miller A. Impact of exposure to war stress on exacerbations of multiple sclerosis. *Ann Neurol.* 2008;64:143–148.
27. Mitsonis CI, Zervas IM, Mitropoulos PA, et al. The impact of stressful life events on risk of relapse in women with multiple sclerosis: a prospective study. *Eur Psychiatry.* 2008;23: 497–504.
28. Koutsogiannopoulos S, Adelson F, Lee V, Andermann F. Stressors at the onset of adult epilepsy: implications for practice. *Epilepsia.* 2008;49:1451–1456.
29. Christensen J, Li J, Vestergaard M, Olsen J. Stress and epilepsy: a population-based cohort study of epilepsy in parents who lost a child. *Epilepsy Behav.* 2007;11:324–328.
30. Moshe S, Shilo M, Chodick G, et al. Occurrence of seizures in association with work-related stress in young male army recruits. *Epilepsia.* 2008;49:1451–1456.
31. Pinikahana J, Dono J. The lived experience of initial symptoms of and factors triggering epileptic seizures. *Epilepsy Behav.* 2009;15:513–520.
32. Thapar A, Kerr M, Harold G. Stress, anxiety, depression, and epilepsy: investigating the relationship between psychological factors and seizures. *Epilepsy Behav.* 2009;14: 134–140.
33. da Silva Sousa P, Lin K, Garzon E, Sakamoto AC, Yacubian EM. Self-perception of factors that precipitate or inhibit seizures in juvenile myoclonic epilepsy. *Seizure.* 2005;14:340–346.
34. Suurmeijer TP, Reuvekamp MF, Aldenkamp BP. Social functioning, psychological functioning, and quality of life in epilepsy. *Epilepsia.* 2001;42:1160–1168.
35. Frucht MM, Quigg M, Schwaner C, Fountain NB. Distribution of seizure precipitants among epilepsy syndromes. *Epilepsia.* 2000;41:1534–1539.
36. Haut SR, Vouyiouklis M, Shinnar S. Stress and epilepsy: a patient perception survey. *Epilepsy Behav.* 2003;4:511–514.
37. Mattson RH. Emotional effects on seizure occurrence. *Adv Neurol.* 1991;55:453–460.
38. Sperling MR, Schilling CA, Glosser D, Tracy JI, Asadi-Pooya AA. Self-perception of seizure precipitants and their relation to anxiety level, depression, and health locus of control in epilepsy. *Seizure.* 2008;17:302–307.
39. Haut SR, Hall CB, Masur J, Lipton RB. Seizure occurrence: precipitants and prediction. *Neurology.* 2007;69:1905–10.
40. Woods RJ, Gruenthal M. Cognition-induced epilepsy associated with specific emotional precipitants. *Epilepsy Behav.* 2006;9:360–362.
41. Bosnjak J, Vukowvic-Bobic M, Mejaski-Bosnjak V. Effect of war on the occurrence of epileptic seizures in children. *Epilepsy Behav.* 2002;3:502–509.
42. Pritchard PB III. The effect of seizures on hormones. *Epilepsia.* 1991;32:S46–S50.

43. Rao ML, Stefan H, Bauer J. Epileptic but not psychogenic seizures are accompanied by simultaneous elevation of serum pituitary hormones and cortisol levels. *Neuroendocrinology*. 1989;49:33–39.

44. Zobel A, Wellmer J, Schulze-Rauschenbach S, et al. Impairment of inhibitory control of the hypothalamic pituitary adrenocortical system in epilepsy. *Eur Arch Psychiatry Clin Neurosci*. 2004;254:303–311.

45. Aroniadou-Anderjaska V, Qashu F, Braga MF. Mechanisms regulating GABAergic inhibitory transmission in the basolateral amygdala: implications for epilepsy and anxiety disorders. *Amino Acids*. 2007;32:305–315.

46. Joels M. Stress, the hippocampus, and epilepsy. *Epilepsia*. 2009;50:586–597.

47. Drugan RC, Basile AS, Ha JH, Ferland RJ. The protective effects of stress control may be mediated by increased brain levels of benzodiazepine receptor agonists. *Brain Res*. 1994;661:127–136.

48. Layne Moore J, Elliott JO, Lu B, Klatte ET, Charyton C. Serious psychological distress among patients with epilepsy based on the 2005 California Health Interview Survey. *Epilepsia*. 2009;50:1077–1084.

49. Pais-Ribero J, da Silva AM, Meneses RF, Falco C. Relationship between optimism, disease variables, and health perception and quality of life in individuals with epilepsy. *Epilepsy Behav*. 2007;11:33–38.

50. Lee SA, Lee SM, No YJ. Factors contributing to depression in patient with epilepsy. *Epilepsia*. 2010;51:1305–1308.

51. Kanner AM. Depression in epilepsy: a complex relation with unexpected consequences. *Curr Opin Neurol*. 2008;21:190–194.

13

Stress Management in Epilepsy

Despite the best efforts of modern medical epilepsy care, many patients have poorly controlled seizures or experience depression or anxiety. Patients and their physicians may try complementary techniques, especially nonpharmacologic ones, to reduce the burden of seizures and to ease anxiety and depression.

Patients with uncontrolled seizures cite stress as one of the most important seizure precipitants (1). Stress management may be accomplished through many techniques, including aerobic exercise, yoga, biofeedback, meditation, massage, and many other methods that can relax the mind and body. Patients often supplement medical treatment with these techniques to combat uncontrolled seizures (1–2). Unfortunately, many patients avoid activities like exercise and yoga for fear of seizure exacerbation and injury. Additionally, social isolation may also reduce participation (3). This chapter explores the potential benefits and risks of stress management techniques for epilepsy.

EXERCISE AND EPILEPSY

The benefits of aerobic and weight-bearing exercises are well established. Exercise improves the course of many chronic illnesses and in some cases prevents them. The signs and symptoms of hyperlipidemia, high blood pressure, obesity, coronary artery disease, osteoporosis, and diabetes are all improved by regular exercise. Exercise remains one of the best established ways to reduce cognitive decline and biomarkers of disease in patients with Alzheimer disease and healthy elderly persons (4–5). However, the benefits of exercise for epilepsy are less well established and, as a result, not routinely recommended by most clinicians.

THE RELATIONSHIP BETWEEN EXERCISE AND SEIZURES

People with epilepsy (PWE) exercise less than the general population (6). Many treating physicians are reluctant to encourage physical exercise because they fear that strenuous exercise and overheating could provoke a seizure or cause physical injury. Several cases of exercise-induced seizures are documented (7–9). Patients with partial or generalized types of epilepsy are at potential risk. Unfortunately, because of the limited number of case studies, we cannot predict an individual's risk for exercise-induced seizures. Also, which exercises induce seizures and how much exercise induces seizures are unknown. Our anecdotal experience is that multiple factors are often involved, including tiredness (e.g., worsened by sleep deprivation), ambient temperature (i.e., exercise in hot temperature is more stressful and more likely to cause a seizure), and duration and intensity of exercise. Further, in some patients, efforts to hydrate with electrolyte solutions (e.g., Gatorade, Hammer Endurolytes) may reduce risk of exercise-induced seizures. It is uncertain if some age groups are more prone to exercise-induced seizures. They may be more common in children, but children may also exercise more frequently than adults. Individuals with sodium channel (SCNIA) mutations are at increased risk of seizures with over heating. It is important to distinguish exercise-induced seizures from paroxysmal kinesiogenic choreoathetosis, a movement disorder that often responds to very low doses of carbamazepine.

Basic science research on exercise and epilepsy is scant. A Brazilian research team studied a rat temporal lobe epilepsy model. The researchers predicted exercise would provoke seizures but found the opposite. Compared with controls (animals that had no physical exercise), animals that did periodic treadmill running had fewer seizures (10).

Deep breathing, hyperventilation, is used to activate abnormal discharges (epileptiform activity) during an electroencephalogram (EEG). This provocative measure is particularly useful to diagnose absence epilepsy of childhood, a condition characterized by brief staring spells with a stereotyped, corresponding EEG abnormality (known as 3-Hz spike and wave). The ability to activate seizures and EEG abnormalities by hyperventilation infers a potential risk of seizures from increased respirations during strenuous exercise in PWE. Some physicians cautioned their patients against exercise based on this rationale. However, one study of children with absence epilepsy concluded that hyperventilation and strenuous exercise are not the same. Although seizures and EEG abnormalities increased during hyperventilation, they did not occur when the children exercised (11). The authors concluded that children with absence epilepsy should not be discouraged from exercising. Additional studies corroborating these findings and extending them to other types of epilepsy are needed.

Clinical Studies of Exercise and Epilepsy

Several small clinical studies examined the effects of exercise on PWE. Denio and colleagues (12) surveyed an epilepsy clinic population as to their exercise habits and concluded that patients who exercised regularly had fewer seizures. After a 4-week program of exercise in 19 patients with uncontrolled seizures, Nakken and colleagues (13) found no increase in seizure frequency associated with the training program, but 6 patients had seizures while exercising. Whether the seizures were random events or were induced by exercise is unclear. In a follow-up study by the same group, 15 women with uncontrolled epilepsy were placed in a 15-week exercise program (14). Seizure frequency for the group decreased significantly during the program compared with baseline seizure frequency. Additional psychological and physical benefits of exercise were documented during the training period.

In a survey of 204 Norwegian PWE, only 10% reported that seizures occurred frequently with exercise, but nearly half of those who exercised regularly experienced at least one seizure associated with exercise. Among patients who commented on the relation between exercise and seizures, approximately one third believed that exercise reduced seizures.

If exercise reduces seizures in some patients, is this the result of a direct effect on the brain? Some suggest that physiologic changes from daily aerobic exercise such as general brain arousal and increased beta-endorphins (naturally occurring opiods or pain relievers present in the brain) may inhibit seizures. However, the effect may also be indirect. Daily aerobic exercise may act as a "stress vaccine," whereby catecholamines (including adrenaline) released in the body during stressful events seem to decrease as physical fitness increases (15). Similar effects may also occur with other stress hormones such as cortisol. A controlled study in patients with congestive heart failure revealed significant improvements in stress management for patients during an exercise program (2). Since mounting evidence supports stress as a provocative factor in some patients' epilepsy, exercise may indirectly reduce seizure frequency.

Potential Benefits of Exercise in Epilepsy

In addition to general health benefits and possible seizure reduction, there are more reasons for PWE to exercise. Many patients use antiepileptic drugs (AEDs) that increase the risk for osteoporosis and bone fractures. Medications such as phenytoin and carbamazepine may interfere with normal vitamin D metabolism and, therefore, with calcium deposition into bone. This effect, especially when combined with a sedentary and indoor lifestyle, is a significant risk for weak bones and possible fractures. The enhanced risk of falling from seizures or from the gait unsteadiness that may result from certain AEDs increases the risk of injury and fractures even more. Studies in patients with osteoporosis document a positive effect of exercise on bone strength (16–17). Thus, exercise may help prevent bone loss in patients taking AEDs.

Mood and anxiety disorders are more common in PWE than the general population (18). Among patients with anxiety and depression who do not have epilepsy, small uncontrolled studies indicate a positive effect of exercise on anxiety and depression (19). We lack large randomized and controlled studies on exercise and psychiatric disorders. Similarly, there are few well-powered studies on the effects of exercise on mood and anxiety in epilepsy, but preliminary studies and surveys are encouraging. Roth and colleagues (20) analyzed self-report measures in 114 PWE and concluded that regular exercise reduced the incidence of depression. Additionally, both exercise and epilepsy studies by the Norwegian group indicated psychological benefits for the patients who exercised (13–14).

Recommendations for Exercise in PWE

Regular exercise can improve physical and mental health. Exercise as a means to reduce seizure frequency or alleviate anxiety and depression in epilepsy remains unproven. However, based on data from individuals without epilepsy and limited data in epilepsy, it is likely that beneficial effects will be realized by most patients. These are best established for cardiovascular and bone health, supported by more limited data for mental health, and least established for seizure control. Exercise programs should be individualized based on the relative risk of seizures and injury because mild to moderate exercise rarely induces seizures. In the initial stages of all exercise programs, intensity should be gradually ramped up in a supervised setting. Patients with frequent seizures that impair consciousness or motor control should choose the safest exercise apparatus available, for instance, a recumbent (low) stationary bicycle instead of a treadmill. In patients with seizures that cause loss of balance, padded or carpeted exercise areas and helmets may be worthwhile. Patients must pay attention to warning signs, such as auras during exercise, as these are opportunities to terminate the exercise and secure a safe position in case of a seizure. Similarly, patients should avoid potentially dangerous exercise, such as open-water swimming, if they are sleep deprived.

Although many patients cannot sustain prolonged strenuous exercise, fortunately, even modest levels of exercise may be beneficial. Among postmenopausal women, those who walked at least 4 hours each week had a 41% lower risk of hip fracture compared with those who walked for less than 1 hour (21). For PWE who are unwilling or unable to exercise and for those patients whose seizures occur frequently with aerobic exercise, other forms of physical fitness such as yoga may be safe and effective alternatives.

Yoga and Epilepsy

Yoga developed in India over the past 5,000 years. It has exploded in popularity to maintain general health, reduce stress, and complement standard medical therapy. Yoga literally means "to yoke together" or to "make whole." There are several types of yoga, but the type most applicable to complementary medicine is hatha yoga and its derivatives. The main components of hatha yoga are meditation, controlled breathing, and physical postures. Although elements of yoga are found in ancient Hindu spiritual texts, practicing yoga is not a religious activity for most people. Many patients need to be reassured that yoga does not conflict with their religious beliefs. Yoga is also not a competitive sport. One need not be a contortionist or gymnast to do it. Therapeutic yoga programs require instructors to be sensitive to the needs and abilities of the individual. Yoga may be practiced at many levels, and patients of all body types, flexibilities, and abilities may derive benefits. Yoga can also be adapted for patients in wheelchairs.

Studies document that yoga is associated with physiologic changes in the musculoskeletal, respiratory, metabolic, cardiovascular, and central nervous systems. These effects can benefit patients with high blood pressure, asthma, and carpal tunnel syndrome (22–25). The effects of yoga on the brain include increased EEG alpha wave activity during yogic breathing and meditation (26). Alpha waves are associated with calm, quiet, and wakefulness. Positron emission tomography scans show changes in cerebral blood flow during meditation (27). These neurophysiologic effects may explain yoga's positive influence on stress management.

Studies of Yoga in Epilepsy

Few studies of yoga and epilepsy have been done. One study looked at yoga in 3 small groups of patients, all with uncontrolled seizures (28). Ten patients were prescribed a 6-month trial of yoga. Another group performed movements that mimicked yoga. The third group performed no movements. Seizure frequency was reduced by 86% in the yoga group, but no change in seizure frequency occurred in the remaining 2 groups. Stress, which was measured by the galvanic skin response, was reduced in the yoga group (29). These results have not been replicated by other investigators.

BENEFITS AND POSSIBLE RISKS

No adverse effects of yoga for epilepsy are documented in the medical literature. In our experience with a supervised program for patients, seizures during yoga classes are rare. When seizures did occur, they occurred in patients new to the program and anxious about the experience. Invariably, patients became more comfortable as they learned yoga. Controlled breathing should be performed gently and slowly to avoid hyperventilation, which can cause seizures in susceptible patients. While joint and musculoskeletal injuries may rarely result from certain yoga postures, they are uncommon with gentle, therapeutic forms of yoga.

BIOFEEDBACK AND NEUROFEEDBACK THERAPY

The Association for Applied Psychophysiology and Biofeedback defines biofeedback as follows:

> A process that enables an individual to learn how to change physiological activity for the purposes of improving health and performance. Precise instruments measure physiological activity such as brainwaves, heart function, breathing, muscle

activity, and skin temperature. These instruments rapidly and accurately 'feed back' information to the user. The presentation of this information—often in conjunction with changes in thinking, emotions, and behavior—supports desired physiological changes. Over time, these changes can endure without continued use of an instrument.

SENSORIMOTOR RHYTHM TRAINING

Neurofeedback therapy (NFT) is biofeedback training that teaches patients to alter their EEG rhythms. In the late 1960s, Sterman and colleagues discovered a 14-Hz EEG rhythm over the sensorimotor cortex in animals, later termed the *sensorimotor rhythm* (SMR)(30). The appearance of the SMR correlated with reduced muscle tension in cats. The animals produced the rhythm in response to a reward. Subsequent animal studies demonstrated a protective effect of the SMR in response to proconvulsants. Over the past few decades, small studies and case reports of patients described improvement in seizure control as well as cognitive and memory performance following SMR training (30–32). Among 63 studies of NFT and epilepsy between 1970 and 2005, 10 studies for medically refractory seizures had adequate outcome data to perform a meta-analysis (33). Weekly seizures were reduced in 64 of 87 patients (74%), an effect considered to be significant even after accounting for the small sample sizes and diverse populations. However, these were not controlled or randomized studies, so patient selection and other biases could have influenced outcome data. Neurofeedback therapy has not gained broad acceptance, most likely owing to the lack of large prospective trials confirming its efficacy, the paucity of trained practitioners, and the significant training commitment required by patients (one to three 1-hour sessions per week for 3 months to 1 year or longer) (34).

Neurofeedback therapy is one of the nontraditional therapies that have great potential. The scientific rationale for its efficacy is demonstrated in animal models. The alternative and traditional medical communities have not systematically studied paradigms that are most effective, nor are there well-powered, randomized and controlled trials to identify methodologies and patient groups who may respond well to this modality. Rather, NFT is often performed by practitioners who have limited training, work in isolation, and have no way to determine what aspect of their results are due to NFT, nonepileptic seizures, medication changes, lifestyle factors, patient selection, investigator bias, patient bias, or other factors.

SLOW CORTICAL POTENTIALS

Some clinicians favor conditioning patients to control slow cortical potentials (SCPs) instead of the SMR. Slow cortical potentials reflect the excitability of the cerebral cortex and therefore the relative risk of seizures. Negative SCPs indicate widespread depolarization in cortical neurons and may correlate with lowered seizure threshold, while positive SCPs reflect decreased cortical excitability and better control of seizures. Antiepileptic drugs diminish negative SCPs (35). Negative SCPs and paroxysmal depolarization shifts in cortical neurons occur simultaneously (36). Conversely, functional magnetic resonance imaging showed deactivation of frontal lobe and thalamic regions in patients who could reliably produce positive SCPs (37). One group of German researchers attributed complete seizure control in 6 of 18 patients with medically refractory epilepsy to mastering control of SCPs (35). A more recent study demonstrated greater than 50% seizure reduction in 14 of 30 patients trained to self-regulate SCPs (38). Treatment successes were correlated with patient ability at the end of the training sessions.

MASSAGE AND AROMATHERAPY

Massage may slow heart rate and brain wave activity along with reducing anxiety levels (39). Along with herbal supplements, massage was the most frequent complementary therapy used by PWE in one survey (40). The widely accepted notion that massage improves general health and reduces tension led health care providers dealing with chronic illness to recommend massage. Thus, massage therapy is a standard addition to conventional medicine at many medical centers treating patients with cancer, chronic pain, asthma, and other disorders. Unfortunately, no controlled studies examine which of the dozens of massage techniques may be effective for reducing stress or seizure activity for PWE.

Aromatherapy was used with massage or hypnotherapy in patients with neurologic and behavioral disorders. Herz (41) reviewed 18 studies of the neuropsychiatric effects of aromatherapy and concluded that odors affect mood and behavior. The largest reported experience of the benefits of aromatherapy in 100 PWE comes from Birmingham University in the United Kingdom. One third of patients became seizure-free for a year after treatment, with effects most notable for those who had aromatherapy combined with hypnosis. Unfortunately, the study was not controlled, and selection bias was present. Additionally, the study highlighted the intense commitment required by patients to maintain treatments.

Meditation

Controversy exists concerning the relative benefits and safety of meditation techniques like transcendental meditation for PWE. One small study of yogic meditation suggested an improvement in seizure control for patients practicing twice-daily meditation for 3 months (42). Larger well-controlled studies are not available to confirm or refute these promising results. While the calming effects of meditation may help most PWE, some researchers question whether meditation may increase seizure activity in some patients (43). During both sleep and EEG activation procedures (hyperventilation and photic stimulation), brain regions synchronize electrically. For susceptible patients like those with primary generalized epilepsy, the synchronization of large cortical regions may provoke seizures. Similarly, the trancelike states induced by meditation may enhance electrical synchrony across brain regions, leading to potential seizures for vulnerable patients. Until more data are available, it is prudent for PWE to learn and practice meditation in a supervised setting.

REFERENCES

1. Ramaratnam S, Sridharan K. Yoga for epilepsy (Cochrane review). In: *The Cochrane Library, Issue 1, 2001*. Oxford, United Kingdom: Update Software; 2001.
2. Luskin F, Reitz M, Newell K, Quinn TG, Haskell W. A controlled pilot study of stress management training of elderly patients with congestive heart failure. *Prev Cardiol*. 2002; 5:168–172.
3. Steinhoff BJ, Neususs K, Thegeder H, Reimers CD. Leisure time activity and physical fitness in patients with epilepsy. *Epilepsia*. 1996;37:1221–1227.
4. Liang KY, Mintun MA, Fagan AM, et al. Exercise and Alzheimer's disease biomarkers in cognitively normal older adults. *Ann Neurol*. 2010;68:311–318.
5. Plassman BL, Williams JW Jr, Burke JR, Holsinger T, Benjamin S. Systematic review: factors associated with risk for and possible prevention of cognitive decline in later life. *Ann Intern Med*. 2010;153:182–193.
6. Jalava M, Sillanpaa M. Physical activity, health-related fitness, and health experience in adults with childhood-onset epilepsy: a controlled study. *Epilepsia*. 1997;38:424–429.
7. Ogunyemi AO, Gomez MR, Klass DW. Seizures induced by exercise. *Neurology*. 1988; 38:633–634.
8. Sturm JW, Fedi M, Berkovic SF, Reutens DC. Exercise-induced temporal lobe epilepsy. *Neurology*. 2002;59:1246–1248.
9. Schmitt B, Thun-Hohenstein L, Vontobel H, Boltshauser E. Seizures induced by physical exercise: report of two cases. *Neuropediatrics*. 1994;25:51–53.
10. Arida RM, Scorza FA, dos Santos NF, Peres CA, Cavalheiro EA. Effect of physical exercise on seizure occurrence in a model of temporal lobe epilepsy in rats. *Epilepsy Res*. 1999;37:45–52.
11. Esquivel E, Chaussain M, Plouin P, Ponsot G, Arthuis M. Phyical exercise and voluntary hyperventilation in childhood absence epilepsy. *Electroencephalogr Clin Neurophysiol*. 1991;79:127–132.
12. Denio LS, Drake ME Jr, Pakalnis A. The effect of exercise on seizure frequency. *J Med*. 1989;20:171–176.
13. Nakken KO, Bjorholt P.G., Johannessen SI, Loyning T, Lind E. Effects of physical training on aerobic capacity, seizure occurrence, and serum level of antiepileptic drugs in adults with epilepsy. *Epilepsia*. 1990;31:88–94.
14. Eriksen HR, Ellertsen B, Gronningsaeter H, Nakken KO, Loyning Y, Ursin H. Physical exercise in women with intractable epilepsy. *Epilepsia*. 1994;35:1256–1264.
15. Nakken KO, Loyning A, Loyning T, Gloersen G, Larsson PG. Does physical exercise influence the occurrence of epileptiform EEG discharges in children? *Epilepsia*. 1997; 38:279–284.
16. Srivastava M, Deal C. Osteoporosis in the elderly: prevention and treatment. *Clin Geriatr Med*. 2002;18:529–555.
17. Luliano-Burns S, Saxon L, Naughton G, Gibbons K, Bass SL. Regional specificity of exercise and calcium during skeletal growth in girls: a randomized controlled trial. *J Bone Miner Res*. 2003;18:156–162.

18. Trimble MR, Perez MM. Quantification of psychopathology in adult patients with epilepsy. In: Kulig B, Meinardi H, Stores G, eds. *Epilepsy and Behavior*. Lisse, Netherlands: Swets and Zeitlinger; 1980:118–126.

19. Dunn AL, Trivedi MH, O'Neal HA. Physical activity dose-response effects on outcomes of depression and anxiety. *Med Sci Sports Exerc*. 2001;33:S587–S597.

20. Roth DL, Goode KT, Williams VL, Faught E. Physical exercise, stressful life experience, and depression in adults with epilepsy. *Epilepsia*. 1994;35:1248–1255.

21. Feskanich D, Willett W, Colditz G. Walking and leisure-time activity and risk of hip fracture in postmenopausal women. *JAMA*. 2002;288:2300–2306.

22. Vempati RP, Telles S. Yoga-based guided relaxation reduces sympathetic activity judged from baseline levels. *Psychol Rep*. 2002;90:487–494.

23. Sundar S, Agrawal SK, Singh VP, Bhattacharya SK, Udupa KN, Vaish SK. Role of yoga in management of essential hypertension. *Acta Cardiol*. 1984;39:203–208.

24. Manocha R, Marks GB, Kenchington P, Peters D, Salome CM. Sahaja yoga in the management of moderate to severe asthma: a randomized controlled trial. *Thorax*. 2002;57: 110–115.

25. Garfinkel MS, Singhal A, Katz WA, Allan DA, Reshetar R, Schumacher HR Jr. Yoga-based intervention for carpal tunnel syndrome: a randomized trial. *JAMA*. 1998;280:1601–1603.

26. Aftanas LI, Golocheikine SA. Human anterior and frontal midline theta and lower alpha reflect emotionally positive state and internalized attention: high-resolution EEG investigation of meditation. *Neurosci Lett*. 2001;310:57–60.

27. Lou HC, Kjaer TW, Friberg L, Wildschiodtz G, Holm S, Nowak M. A 15O-H2O PET study of meditation and the resting state of normal consciousness. *Hum Brain Mapp*. 1999;7:98–105.

28. Panjwani U, Selvamurthy W, Singh SH, Gupta HL, Thakur L, Rai UC. Effect of Sahaja yoga practice on seizure control and EEG changes in patients with epilepsy. *Indian J Med Res*. 1996;103:165–172.

29. Panjwani U, Gupta HL, Singh SH, Selvamurthy W, Rai UC. Effect of Sahaja yoga practice on stress management in patients of epilepsy. *Indian J Physiol Pharmacol*. 1995; 39:111–116.

30. Sterman MB. Biofeedback in the treatment of epilepsy. *Cleve Clin J Med*. 2010;77.

31. Seifert AR, Lubar JF. Reduction of epileptic seizures through EEG biofeedback training. *Biol Psychol*. 1975;3:157–184.

32. Vernon D, Egner T, Cooper N, et al. The effect of training distinct neurofeedback protocols on aspects of cognitive performances. *Int J Psychophysiol*. 2003;47:75–85.

33. Tan G, Thornby J, Hammond DC, et al. Meta-analysis of EEG biofeedback in treating epilepsy. *Clin EEG Neurosci*. 2009;40:173–179.

34. Sterman MB, Friar L. Suppression of seizures in an epileptic following sensorimotor EEG feedback training. *Electroencephalogr Clin Neurophysiol*. 1972;33:89–95.

35. Rockstroh B, Elbert T, Birbaumer N, et al. Cortical self-regulation in patients with epilepsy. *Epilepsy Res*. 1993;14:63–72.

36. Ikeda A, Terada K, Mikuni N, et al. Subdural recording of ictal DC shifts in neocortical seizures in humans. *Epilepsia*. 1996;37:662–674.

37. Strehl U, Trevorrow T, Veit R, et al. Deactivation of brain areas during self-regulation of slow cortical potentials in seizure patients. *Appl Psychophysiol Biofeedback*. 2006;31: 85–94.

38. Strehl U, Kotchoubey B, Trevorrow T, Birbaumer N. Predictors of seizure reduction after self-regulation of slow cortical potentials as a treatment of drug-resistant epilepsy. *Epilepsy Behav*. 2005;6:156–166.

39. Diego MA, Field T, Sanders C, Hernandez-Reif M. Massage therapy of moderate and light pressure and vibrator effects on EEG and heart rate. *Int J Neurosci*. 2004;114:31–44.

40. Peebles CT, McAuley JW, Roach J, Moore JL, Reeves AL. Alternative medicine use by patients with epilepsy. *Epilepsy Behav.* 2000;1:74–77.

41. Herz RS. Aromatherapy facts and fictions: a scientific analysis of olfactory effects on mood, physiology and behavior. *Int J Neurosci.* 2009;119:263–290.

42. Rajesh B, Jayachandran D, Mohandas G, Radhakrishnan K. A pilot study of a yoga meditation protocol for patients with medically refractory epilepsy. *J Altern Complement Med.* 2006;12:367–371.

43. Lansky EP, St Louis EK. Transcendental meditation: a double-edged sword in epilepsy? *Epilepsy Behav.* 2006;9:394–400.

14

Sleep and Seizures

Good-quality sleep is important for physical and mental health as well as cognitive function. Very poor sleep on a single night or mildly to moderately impaired sleep over many days can cause daytime sleepiness, mood disturbances, trouble concentrating, difficulty with memory, and, for people with epilepsy (PWE), an increased risk of seizures. There are many reasons for inadequate sleep in people with or without epilepsy, which include a stressful lifestyle; a bedroom that is noisy, hot/cold, or bright; an uncomfortable mattress; pain; mood disorders such as depression and anxiety (see Chapter 11); medical conditions; and sleep disorders.

Some sleep disorders increase the risk of seizures during the day or night because they disrupt sleep. In contrast, nighttime seizures and antiepileptic drug (AED) side effects can interfere with restorative sleep, so some PWE find themselves in an unfortunate cycle of sleep disruption leading to seizures and further sleep disruption.

The daytime sleepiness and trouble with thinking may be particularly problematic in PWE who struggle with sleepiness and trouble thinking from AEDs or their seizures (1–2). The resulting impact on quality of life, school and work performance, and activities such as driving can be substantial. Approximately two thirds of PWE complain of feeling sleepy during the day, one third have difficulty falling asleep or staying asleep, and more blame sleep difficulties for problems at work (1, 3–4).

This chapter discusses the relationships between sleep, sleep disorders, and seizures, and then outlines the use of complementary therapies on sleep problems.

RELATIONSHIPS BETWEEN SLEEP, SLEEP DISORDERS, AND SEIZURES

Sleep is an active process involving different brain networks. Sleep is organized into non–rapid eye movement (NREM) sleep (subdivided into 4 stages) and rapid

185

eye movement (REM) sleep (when dreaming occurs). Each night, there are multiple 90-minute cycles during which NREM and REM sleep occur in a specific sequence. *Sleep organization* refers to the degree to which cycles of NREM and REM sleep occur in normal sequential patterns throughout the night. This can be evaluated in someone with an overnight sleep test, also called polysomnography, which uses electroencephalography (EEG), eye movements, respiratory function, and muscle movement to determine when the stages of NREM and REM sleep occur and in what sequence. During REM sleep, for example, there are no movements of the arms and legs, but there are intermittent and rapid movements of the eyes.

EFFECTS OF SEIZURES ON SLEEP

Having a seizure during sleep can disrupt sleep organization. Seizures can wake the person up or replace deep sleep with light sleep. Normal sleep may not return until the aftereffects of the seizure (the postictal state) are over.

There are many seizures that can occur during the night. These include the spectrum of partial and generalized seizures, and some that are only diagnosed with a sleep EEG (e.g., Landau-Kleffner syndrome, continuous spikes and waves during sleep, and electrical status epilepticus in sleep) (5–6). Among partial-onset seizures, those of the frontal lobes are particularly likely to occur during sleep, including the subgroup with autosomal-dominant nocturnal frontal lobe epilepsy. Partial seizures during sleep usually occur during NREM sleep (6). Children with benign rolandic epilepsy often have seizures around the time of sleep onset or offset. In these children, epileptiform activity on EEG is dramatically increased during NREM sleep. Among those with generalized epilepsy, those with juvenile myoclonic epilepsy and generalized tonic-clonic seizures on awakening are especially prone to seizures within an hour after awakening. People with epilepsy whose seizures tend to occur shortly after awakening are often very sensitive to alcohol withdrawal.

Tonic-clonic seizures in sleep nearly always affect sleep organization. Studying the effect of tonic-clonic seizures on sleep in 77 PWE, researchers found reduced total sleep time, less REM sleep than normal, increased time awake after sleep onset, and increased light sleep all during the night when a seizure occurred (7). Another study of 11 PWE with temporal lobe seizures found similar disruptions of sleep organization during nights when seizures occurred, including reduced REM and deep NREM sleep compared with expected levels (8). In addition, the PWE were sleepier during the day following their nighttime seizures. This is interesting because, for some PWEs who have seizures during sleep, the only clue that they may have had a seizure during the previous night is feeling unusually tired during the day. Seizures during the day can also decrease REM sleep that night (9).

Whether a person has partial-onset or tonic-clonic seizures, sleep organization after a seizure-free day and during seizure-free nights should generally be normal unless there are other reasons not to get a good night's sleep, such as a sleep disorder.

EFFECTS OF SLEEP DISORDERS ON SEIZURES

Sleep disorders are medical conditions that affect the duration, quality, and/or restorative nature of sleep. The most common sleep disorders in PWE are sleep apnea, insomnia, periodic limb movements, and restless legs syndrome (RLS). Each can disrupt sleep organization and cause excessive daytime sleepiness, and one—sleep apnea—causes a temporary drop in blood oxygen levels. Each of these disorders could potentially increase the risk of seizures in PWE.

Sleep apnea is distinguished by repetitive periods of a lack of breathing during sleep, called *apneas*, lasting for 10 or more seconds. During apneas, the amount of oxygen in the blood drops (called *desaturation*), and the affected individual may then awaken or quickly transition from deep to light sleep (called *arousals*) as often as 100 times per hour or more, though they may have no memory of this. Sleep organization is often severely disrupted.

There are 2 types of sleep apnea: obstructive and central. Obstructive sleep apnea (OSA) is more common than central sleep apnea and is caused by some form of obstruction at the back of the throat or the upper part of the airway, which may be apparent only when the throat muscles relax during sleep. Persons with OSA are often overweight and may have large or thick necks, and they usually snore loudly. During their apneas, persons with OSA appear to be struggling to breathe but are unable to move air because of the obstruction, until they arouse enough to have more voluntary control over the upper-airway muscles, thereby relieving the obstruction. Obstructive sleep apnea is diagnosed with a polysomnogram.

About 2% of women and 4% of men have OSA, defined as excessive daytime sleepiness and at least 5 apneas per hour of sleep (10). Obstructive sleep apnea may occur even more frequently in PWE, and in these persons, the successful treatment of OSA can result in an improvement in seizure frequency (3, 11–13).

Central sleep apnea also causes frequent apneas during the night and arousals but without the apparent attempts to breathe, as seen in those with OSA, and also without snoring. Central sleep apnea is usually a symptom of a brain abnormality.

Insomnia refers to difficulty falling asleep or difficulty staying asleep, combined with daytime sleepiness or impairment of daytime performance. To be considered a sleep disorder, insomnia usually must persist for weeks to months since it is quite common for otherwise healthy persons to have occasional trouble falling or staying asleep.

There are many causes of insomnia, including environmental, dietary, or behavioral factors (noisy bedroom, uncomfortable bed, ingesting caffeine in the evening, strenuous exercise before bedtime); mood disorders (anxiety or depression); stress; pain; medications with stimulating properties taken at bedtime (lamotrigine); shift work or travel (jet lag); and medical conditions (coughing, kidney problems, and heart failure).

Insomnia occurs more often in PWE than in the general population (1, 14). Trouble falling asleep might suggest an associated mood disorder (see Chapter 11), stress, a stimulating seizure medication, or recently discontinued sedating seizure medication. Trouble staying asleep might be indicative of seizures, as discussed earlier.

Periodic limb movements are characterized by frequent, brief, and repetitive leg movements during sleep. These movements may disrupt sleep organization and be associated with arousals as seen on polysomnography. When leg movements are particularly prominent, there may be associated excessive daytime sleepiness or insomnia. Patients may be unaware of the movements, but bed partners usually note them. Periodic limb movements and RLS may occur in otherwise healthy people but can also be seen in persons with kidney disease, circulatory problems in the legs, low hematocrit levels, nerve-related pain in the legs, various other causes of pain, and caffeine (15).

Persons with RLS experience an unpleasant crawling or aching sensation in the legs that precipitates and is improved by moving the legs. Restless legs syndrome occurs at night in association with periodic leg movements as well as during the day while affected persons are sitting or lying down. Restless legs syndrome may occur more commonly in PWEs than in the general population (1).

COMPLEMENTARY THERAPIES FOR SLEEP PROBLEMS

Sleep disorders are potentially serious medical illnesses that should be evaluated by physicians with the appropriate training and background to recommend therapy when medically necessary and monitor the response to therapy. Referral to a sleep center for further evaluation and possible polysomnography is often required to correctly diagnose the problem.

Therefore, before PWE consider complementary approaches to treat apparent problems with their sleep, they should seek appropriate medical evaluation and care. Some sleep disorders, such as OSA, significantly increase the risk of cardiovascular problems such as heart attack and stroke. A discussion of therapies for sleep disorders is beyond the scope of this chapter. However, before any treatment is started, whether conventional or complementary and alternative medicine (CAM), the physician should assess whether nighttime seizures may be a factor since this may be amenable to a change in AEDs. This evaluation may require nighttime video EEG monitoring. Also, the physician should determine whether stimulating AEDs (such as lamotrigine and felbamate) are being taken close to bedtime and should encourage PWE to adopt good sleep habits (see Table 14.1) to see if sleep-related problems improve. For example, while moderate exercise is important for general health benefits in PWE, exercise late in the evening can cause trouble falling asleep. Also, while some AEDs such

Table 14.1   Tips for Getting a Good Night's Sleep[a]

General	Go to sleep at about the same time each night and awaken at the same time each morning. Wide fluctuations between workdays and days off can further impair your sleep.
	Try not to nap. If you do, restrict this to about an hour per day and do it relatively early (before 4 in the afternoon).
	If you are not sleepy, either do not go to bed or arise from bed. Do quiet, relaxing activities until you feel sleepy, then return to bed.
	Avoid doing stimulating, frustrating, or anxiety-provoking activities in bed or in the bedroom (watching television, studying, balancing the checkbook, etc). Try to reserve the bedroom and especially the bed for sleep and sexual activity.
Use of drugs	Avoid coffee, tea, cola, or other caffeinated beverages after about noon. Also avoid chocolate late in the day.
	If you smoke, avoid this in the hour or two before bedtime.
	If you drink alcohol, limit this to 1–2 drinks per day and do not drink immediately before bedtime. Although you may find this relaxing, alcohol actually can interfere with sleep later in the night.
	If you take prescription drugs or over-the-counter drugs that can be stimulating, discuss dosing times with your doctor.
Exercise	Exercise, particularly aerobic exercise, is good for both sleep and overall health and should be encouraged.
	Avoid stimulating exercise in the evening (do this at least 5 hours before bedtime).
Bedtime ritual	Perform relaxing activities in the hour before bedtime.
	Make sure your sleeping environment is as comfortable as possible, paying attention to temperature, noise, and light.
	Do not eat a heavy meal just before bedtime, although a light snack might help induce drowsiness.
	It is sometimes helpful to place paper and pen by the bedside. If you find yourself worrying about completing or remembering a task the next day, write it down and let it go.
During the night	If you awaken and find you cannot get back to sleep, arise from bed and do quiet, relaxing activities until you are drowsy, then return to bed.
	Place clocks so that the time is not visible from the bed.

[a]Reproduced from (38).

as levetiracetam are often neither sedating nor stimulating, they may in some individuals—especially children—cause insomnia (16).

Few research studies have evaluated the safety and effectiveness of complementary treatments for sleep-related problems or particular sleep disorders specifically in PWE, and studies in other populations have generally focused only on insomnia and, in particular, on the length of time it takes to fall asleep, total sleep duration, and the quality of sleep.

NEUROBEHAVIORAL APPROACHES

Neurobehavioral approaches are a form of CAM therapy referred to as mind-body medicine. They are intended to promote relaxation and enhance the mind's ability to influence bodily function and modify how the body and mind respond to stress (17). Mind-body medicine is the most common CAM used by adults with chronic neurologic conditions and includes deep breathing exercises (19%), meditation (13%), and yoga (7%) (18–19). Neurobehavioral approaches for control of seizures are discussed in Chapter 6 and for treatment of depression and anxiety in Chapter 11.

A variety of neurobehavioral approaches can treat insomnia, with cognitive behavioral therapy (CBT) as the most extensively studied (20). Cognitive behavioral therapy has similar benefits for the treatment of insomnia as those of sleep medications in persons with or without medical or mood disorders, including elderly persons (21). In this context, CBT usually provides persons with training on the following: (a) maximizing preparation for sleep and the bedroom as an appropriate environment for sleeping (see Table 14.1), such as limiting caffeine and alcohol in the evening, exercising daily, establishing a quiet and dark bedroom at a comfortable temperature, going to sleep only when sleepy, getting out of bed if unable to sleep, setting a regular morning wake time, and avoiding daytime napping; (b) relaxation therapy; and (c) cognitive therapy to target worries, such as not functioning well due to sleepiness (22).

Studies of mindfulness-based stress reduction for the treatment of insomnia suggest a possible benefit but are viewed as inconclusive because of issues in how the studies were conducted (23). Likewise, hypnosis, either alone or in combination with CBT, appears to be safe and effective, but the available published studies are not definitive (24).

BIOLOGICALLY BASED PRACTICES

Biologically based practices are another subset of CAM therapies and include the use of substances found in nature, such as herbs, foods, vitamins, and animal compounds. This group of practices was the most commonly used form of CAM by the U.S. general population in a 2007 survey (25). The use of herb-derived products by PWE is discussed in Chapter 2 (Herbal Remedies), and herbal remedies for depression and anxiety are outlined in Chapter 11.

No research has specifically studied the efficacy of herbal medicines for sleep-related problems in PWE. One of the most studied herbal medicines for insomnia in the general population is valerian, a flowering plant widely used in Europe and available in the United States as a dietary supplement (26). Reviews of published studies suggest a possible benefit of valerian alone or in combination with hops in the treatment of primary insomnia, though study design issues significantly limit conclusions, and other researchers are not convinced of valerian's effectiveness (26–28). Evidence for homeopathic medicines, either taken alone or in combinations, is lacking (29). Finally, limited studies evaluating the amino acid L-tryptophan and the herbal medicine kava have found suggestive but inconclusive improvements in insomnia (30).

Melatonin is a hormone normally made by the pineal gland. This gland is located deep inside the brain and helps to regulate daily biorhythms, also known as circadian rhythms. Most melatonin is produced by the pineal gland at night and is believed to cause the drowsiness that precedes sleep. Melatonin is also available over the counter as a dietary supplement. In some clinical studies of melatonin as treatment for insomnia, study patients fell asleep sooner, though the difference compared with placebo was modest (31). Melatonin has also been used by shift workers to maintain regular sleep-wake cycles and by travelers to lessen jet lag, and clinical evidence appears to support these effects (32).

Melatonin is among the most popular dietary supplements for PWE (33). There is some suggestive evidence, for example, in one study of children with severe epilepsy, that it may have anticonvulsant properties (34). However, other studies suggest it may worsen seizures in neurologically disabled children and increase EEG abnormalities in persons with temporal lobe epilepsy (35).

People with epilepsy who try one or more of these natural products should inform their physician since these could affect the blood levels of other medications, including AEDs, and may cause side effects that the physician might otherwise attribute to AEDs.

OTHER APPROACHES

Yoga, tai chi (36), massage, and aromatherapy have been used to treat insomnia, including in elderly persons, but published evidence for benefits and safety from studies using generally accepted principles of clinical research is generally lacking (30, 37).

CONCLUSION

People with epilepsy whose seizures are not fully controlled or who experience excessive levels of drowsiness that interfere with daytime functioning should undergo a medical evaluation to see if they may have a sleep disorder. The interrelationships between sleep, sleep disorders, medical and mood disorders, seizures, and seizure medications are complicated, but in any individual PWE, testing such as polysomnography or video EEG monitoring may be helpful to sort out the situation. Doing so may possibly lead to treatments that can potentially improve the quality of sleep, daytime functioning, and even seizure frequency. Many complementary approaches to treat insomnia have been tried and evaluated in studies, most often in people without epilepsy. Neurobehavioral approaches such as CBT appear to be beneficial and safe. However, convincing evidence for the effectiveness of other CAM approaches is not presently available, largely because the ways the studies were conducted are not adequate to reach firm conclusions. Additional research will hopefully further clarify whether any of these treatments work for PWE with sleep disorders and, if they do, who is most likely to benefit.

REFERENCES

1. de Weerd A, de Haas S, Otte A, et al. Subjective sleep disturbance in patients with partial epilepsy: a questionnaire-based study on prevalence and impact on quality of life. *Epilepsia*. 2004;45:1397–1404.
2. Xu X, Brandenburg NA, McDermott AM, Bazil CW. Sleep disturbances reported by refractory partial-onset epilepsy patients receiving polytherapy. *Epilepsia*. 2006;47:1176–1183.
3. Malow BA, Bowes RJ, Lin X. Predictors of sleepiness in epilepsy patients. *Sleep*. 1997;20:1105–1110.
4. Miller M, Vaughn B, Messenheimer J. Subjective sleep quality in patients with epilepsy. *Epilepsia*. 1996;36:43.
5. Loddenkemper T, Fernandez IS, Peters JM. Continuous spike and waves during sleep and electrical status epilepticus in sleep. *J Clin Neurophysiol*. 2011;28:154–164.
6. Bazil CW. Nocturnal seizures. *Semin Neurol*. 2004;24:293–300.
7. Touchon J, Baldy-Moulinier M, Besset A, Cadilhac J. Sleep organization and epilepsy In: Degen R, Rodin E, eds. *Epilepsy, Sleep, and Sleep Deprivation*. 2nd ed. New York, NY: Elsevier; 1991:73–81.
8. Castro L, Bazil C, Walczak T. Nocturnal seizures disrupt sleep architecture and decrease sleep efficiency. *Epilepsia*. 1997;38:49.
9. Bazil CW, Castro LH, Walczak TS. Reduction of rapid eye movement sleep by diurnal and nocturnal seizures in temporal lobe epilepsy. *Arch Neurol*. 2000;57:363–368.
10. Young T, Palta M, Dempsey J, Skatrud J, Weber S, Badr S. The occurrence of sleep-disordered breathing among middle-aged adults. *N Engl J Med*. 1993;328:1230–1235.
11. Beran RG, Plunkett MJ, Holland GJ. Interface of epilepsy and sleep disorders. *Seizure*. 1999;8:97–102.
12. Malow BA, Fromes GA, Aldrich MS. Usefulness of polysomnography in epilepsy patients. *Neurology*. 1997;48:1389–1394.
13. Devinsky O, Ehrenberg B, Barthlen GM, Abramson HS, Luciano D. Epilepsy and sleep apnea syndrome. *Neurology*. 1994;44:2060–2064.
14. Bazil CW. Sleep disturbance in epilepsy patients. *Curr Neurol Neurosci Rep*. 2005;5: 297–298.
15. Trenkwalder C, Walters A, Hening W. Periodic limb movements and restless legs syndrome. *Neurol Clin*. 1996;14:629–650.
16. Perry MS, Benatar M. Efficacy and tolerability of levetiracetam in children younger than 4 years: a retrospective review. *Epilepsia*. 2007;48:1123–1127.
17. Dusek JA, Benson H. Mind-body medicine: a model of comparative clinical impact of the acute stress and relaxation responses. *Minn Med*. 2009;92:47–50.

18. Wells RE, Phillips RS, Schachter SC, McCarthy EP. Complementary and alternative medicine use among U.S. adults with common neurological conditions. *J Neurol.* 2010;257: 1822–1831.

19. Wells RE, Phillips RS, McCarthy EP. Patterns of mind-body therapies in adults with common neurological conditions. *Neuroepidemiology.* 2011;36:46–51.

20. Ebben MR, Spielman AJ. Non-pharmacological treatments for insomnia. *J Behav Med.* 2009;32:244–254.

21. Joshi S, Nonpharmacologic therapy for insomnia in the elderly. *Clin Geriatr Med.* 2008;24:107–119.

22. Siebern AT, Manber R. Insomnia and its effective non-pharmacologic treatment. *Med Clin North Am.* 2010;94:581–591.

23. Winbush NY, Gross CR, Kreitzer MJ. The effects of mindfulness-based stress reduction on sleep disturbance: a systematic review. *Explore.* 2007;3:585–591.

24. Graci GM, Hardie JC. Evidenced-based hypnotherapy for the management of sleep disorders. *Int J Clin Exp Hypn.* 2007;55:288–302.

25. Barnes PM, Bloom B, Nahin RL. Complementary and alternative medicine use among adults and children: United States, 2007. *Natl Health Stat Report.* 2008;10:1–23.

26. Bent S, Padula A, Moore D, Patterson M, Mehling W. Valerian for sleep: a systematic review and meta-analysis. *Am J Med.* 2006;119:1005–1012.

27. Salter S, Brownie S. Treating primary insomnia—the efficacy of valerian and hops. *Aust Fam Physician.* 2010;39:433–437.

28. Taibi DM, Landis CA, Petry H, Vitiello MV. A systematic review of valerian as a sleep aid: safe but not effective. *Sleep Med Rev.* 2007;11:209–230.

29. Cooper KL, Relton C. Homeopathy for insomnia: summary of additional RCT published since systematic review. *Sleep Med Rev.* 2010;14:411.

30. Sarris J, Byrne GJ. A systematic review of insomnia and complementary medicine. *Sleep Med Rev.* 2011;15:99–106.

31. Buscemi N, Vandermeer B, Hooton N, et al. The efficacy and safety of exogenous melatonin for primary sleep disorders. A meta-analysis. *J Gen Intern Med.* 2005;20:1151–1158.

32. Larzelere MM, Campbell JS, Robertson M. Complementary and alternative medicine usage for behavioral health indications. *Prim Care Clin Office Pract.* 2010;37:213–236.

33. Ekstein D, Schachter SC. Natural products in epilepsy—the present situation and perspectives for the future. *Pharmaceuticals.* 2010;3:1426–1445.

34. Peled N, Shorer Z, Peled E, Pillar G. Melatonin effect on seizures in children with severe neurologic deficit disorders. *Epilepsia.* 2001;42:1208–1210.

35. Banach M, Gurdziel E, Jedrych M, Borowicz KK. Melatonin in experimental seizures and epilepsy. *Pharmacol Rep.* 2011;63:1–11.

36. Kuramoto AM. Therapeutic benefits of tai chi exercise: research review. *Wis Med J.* 2006;105:42–46.

37. Gooneratne NS. Complementary and alternative medicine for sleep disturbances in older adults. *Clin Geriatr Med.* 2008;24:121–138.

38. Bazil C. Sleep. In: Schachter SC, Holmes GL, Trenite DGAK, eds. Behavioral Aspects of Epilepsy. Principles & Practice. New York, NY: Demos Medical Publishing; 2008:491.

15

Over-the-Counter Drugs, Alcohol, and Recreational Drugs

The most commonly consumed drugs are not prescribed by physicians but are electively consumed by people for ailments and enjoyment. Over-the-counter (OTC) drugs, alcohol, and recreational drugs can influence seizure activity. The vast majority of OTC drugs are safe for people with epilepsy. While some OTC and recreational drugs make seizures more likely to occur because they interact with antiepileptic drugs (AEDs), most alter the seizure threshold directly. Unfortunately, most drugs that alter the seizure threshold lower it and make seizures more likely to occur. Some, like marijuana, are reported by some patients and by limited data to improve seizure control. However, the data are preliminary and inconclusive.

Seizures can occur for the first time or a breakthrough seizure may occur in someone with well-controlled epilepsy after using an antihistamine or cold/sinus/ allergy medication. The challenge is quantifying risk. Which is more likely to provoke a seizure, taking an OTC allergy medication such as loratadine (Claritin) or experiencing sleep deprivation from severe allergies? Nonsedating antihistamines like loratadine have limited entry into the brain and therefore should have a much lower risk of provoking a seizure than sedating antihistamines, such as diphenhydramine (Bendaryl). Severe sleep deprivation is probably worse. However, loratadine with pseudoephedrine (Claritin-D) has a higher risk of provoking a seizure because of the pseudoephedrine.

Defining risk and benefit is often something that can best be done by a collaboration of patient and physician. It is essential that the cumulative, and sometimes exponential, effect of risk factors is understood. For someone with well-controlled epilepsy who takes antiepileptic medications as prescribed, sleeps well, has little stress, and consumes no alcohol, an antihistamine or decongestant will rarely provoke a seizure. By contrast, if these medications are taken when antiepileptic medications have been missed and the person is sleep deprived and under stress, then the risk of a breakthrough seizure is much higher. If all these risk factors are present, and a seizure-provoking drug is taken, the risk of a seizure increases dramatically.

OVER-THE-COUNTER DRUGS

Some drugs that can be bought without a physician's prescription can lower the seizure threshold, thereby increasing the tendency of someone with epilepsy to have a seizure. This rarely provokes a person's first seizure (Table 15.1). It is hard to determine the frequency with which these medications affect the seizure threshold since the association is often uncertain. For instance, patients take these medications when they have viral illnesses or are simultaneously exposed to other seizure-provoking factors (e.g., sleep deprivation, missed medications). A coincidental seizure may be mistaken for a medication-induced seizure. There are no case-control studies to establish the frequency of seizures associated with OTC medicines. However, many cases of seizures occurring shortly after taking a medication in patients with well-controlled epilepsy or without prior seizures as well as animal models strongly suggest that these drugs can lower the seizure threshold.

Table 15.1   Selected Over-the-Counter Drugs and Foods That Can Affect Seizure Control or Drug Side Effects

Drug/Food	Effect	Common Product[a]
Acetaminophen	Slight decrease in lamotrigine level	Alka-Seltzer
		Drixoral
		Excedrin
		Midol
		Robitussin
		Sudafed
		TheraFlu
		Tylenol
Aspirin or other salicylates[b]	Slight decrease in phenytoin total level but slight increase in phenytoin free level	Alka-Seltzer
	May increase levels of valproate in the blood	Anacin
		Bayer Aspirin
		Bufferin
		Excedrin

Table 15.1   (*continued*)

Diphenhydramine	Can lower seizure threshold (minimum conditions necessary to produce a seizure)	Alka-Seltzer
		PM Pain Benadryl
		· Nytol
		Sominex
Grapefruit juice	Increase in carbamazepine level in the blood, causing side effects	
Phenylephrine	Potential to lower seizure threshold	Dimetapp Cold Drops
		Tylenol Sinus
		DayQuil
Pseudoephedrine	Potential to lower seizure threshold	Sudafed
		Drixoral

[a]These are not all-inclusive lists. Refer to ingredient lists when determining whether a product may affect seizure control or contribute to side effects of drugs.

[b]Low to moderate daily dosages of aspirin (less than 1500 mg/d) are generally very safe for people who take antiepileptic drugs. Higher doses should be taken only after discussion with a physician, especially if phenytoin or valproate is used. Aspirin-free versions of some products listed are available.

Commonly used medications that can lower the seizure threshold include cold, sleep, and allergy preparations that contain antihistamines and decongestants. First-generation antihistamines such as diphenhydramine (Benadryl, Tylenol PM), chlorpheniramine (Chlor-Trimeton), and hydroxyzine (Atarax) block histamine 1 receptors and are mainly used to treat allergies and induce sleep and less often to prevent vomiting or treat motion sickness, vertigo, and cough. The drugs may be abused occasionally as they can relieve opioid-induced itching or potentiate depressant effects of alcohol and other drugs. Second-generation antihistamines such as fexofenadine (Allegra), loratadine (Claritin), cetirizine (Zyrtec), and desloratadine (Clarinex) have lower penetration across the blood-brain barrier, thereby decreasing the risk of seizures as well as sedation.

Decongestants for runny and stuffed noses (rhinitis) may contain pseudoephedrine or phenylephrine. These drugs have a small potential to cause seizures and should be avoided. Anecdotal observations suggest that such seizures induced by these medications may be more common among patients with primary generalized epilepsy. Diphenhydramine ointment applied to the skin for itching appears safe for people with epilepsy.

For aches, pains, and fevers, acetaminophen (e.g., Tylenol) and ibuprofen (e.g., Motrin, Advil) are safe. Ibuprofen can increase blood levels of phenytoin and possibly cause side effects. Aspirin does not affect seizure threshold, but it should not be given to young children. Drug interactions may cause side effects if aspirin is taken by persons with high blood levels of valproate or phenytoin. Propoxyphene, another pain reliever in OTC preparations, can increase carbamazepine levels and cause side effects. Finally, acetaminophen can slightly lower lamotrigine levels, but the clinical relevance of this interaction is uncertain.

ALCOHOL

Alcohol use by people with epilepsy is controversial. Occasional small intake is safe for most adults with epilepsy. Small intake is defined as no more than 2 alcoholic drinks (1 drink = 5 oz wine, 12 oz beer, or 1.5 oz of 80-proof liquor) over 24 hours; if 2 drinks are consumed, it should be with food and spread out over at least 2 to 3 hours. Moderate to heavy alcohol consumption is never recommended for people with epilepsy. Excess alcohol consumption can adversely affect sleep quality, increase medication noncompliance, and cause a withdrawal state that lowers the seizure threshold. The risk of withdrawal seizures markedly increases after consuming 2 or more alcoholic drinks, but some experience withdrawal seizures after fewer drinks.

Intoxication

Alcohol is a central nervous system depressant with pharmacologic properties similar to the general anesthetics. Acute intoxication causes cognitive impairment, emotional lability, nystagmus, dysarthria, and ataxia; stupor, coma, and death can occur. Jackson (1) recognized that higher cortical centers are first affected by alcohol; this initial depression of inhibitory centers can transiently stimulate (or disinhibit) behavior. Blood alcohol levels of 500 mg/dL are lethal in approximately 50% of patients owing to respiratory depression. Concomitant use of other central nervous system depressants (e.g., benzodiazepines) potentiates alcohol intoxication. Seizures can rarely occur during acute intoxication, but animal and human studies suggest that short-term administration of alcohol has antiepileptic properties. Therefore, seizures during intoxication should be thoroughly investigated to exclude other causes.

Withdrawal

Alcohol withdrawal can lower the seizure threshold in patients who occasionally binge-drink or in those who chronically abuse alcohol and are physically dependent. Signs and symptoms of alcohol withdrawal include fine tremor, irritability, and insomnia in mild cases; in more severely affected subjects, lateral nystagmus (opposite the direction of the nystagmus during intoxication), sensory illusions and hallucinations, tremulousness, anorexia, nausea, vomiting, anxiety, tachycardia, and diaphoresis may occur. Delirium tremens is the most serious complication of alcohol withdrawal, occurring in 5% of hospitalized alcoholics, and is fatal in 10% of cases.

Alcohol withdrawal seizures typically occur between 4 and 60 hours after the cessation of drinking. Withdrawal seizures are most common among persons who have abused alcohol for years or in adolescents or young adults who binge-drink. When alcohol consumption stops suddenly or is markedly reduced over a short time, a withdrawal seizure may occur. When seizures occur only in the setting of alcohol withdrawal, they are usually termed "provoked seizures" rather than true epilepsy. Yet those individuals often have an increased susceptibility to epileptic seizures. Similarly, abrupt withdrawal of barbiturates or benzodiazepines can provoke withdrawal seizures.

Treatment of alcohol withdrawal seizures must be individualized. Therapy differs for the college student with known epilepsy who binge-drinks and has a single tonic-clonic seizure 24 hours later and the chronic alcoholic who has a convulsion with other signs of delirium tremens. For the binge-drinking student with epilepsy, if the seizure was witnessed, there is no head injury, and a reliable person can attend to the patient, there is not necessarily a need to come into the hospital. Evidence of missed AEDs should be sought. An oral benzodiazepine may be sufficient. For the chronic alcoholic with signs of sympathetic overactivity, admission is essential, with administration of parenteral benzodiazepines as well as careful evaluation of fluid, electrolyte, nutrition, and neurologic status.

Alcoholism

Individuals with epilepsy are less likely to use or abuse alcohol than the general population. This likely reflects a combination of experience that excess consumption can cause seizures as well as warnings by physicians and pharmacists. Since many AEDs have similar side effects to alcohol (e.g., tiredness, unsteadiness, slurred speech, blurred or double vision, tiredness, impaired coordination), use of alcohol with AEDs can make a person more prone to these adverse effects. Chronic alcoholism is associated with neurologic issues, such as recurrent head injury, cerebral atrophy, and nutritional deficiencies, which may make seizures more likely. Seizures usually occur in individuals who have abused alcohol for at least 10 years, suggesting that long-term neuronal changes (e.g., kindling) or structure (e.g., loss of inhibitory neurons from metabolic deficiencies, cortical scars from head trauma) are required for seizures to develop in people who abuse alcohol but have no other predisposing factors for epilepsy.

ALCOHOL: PHARMACOKINETICS AND EFFECTS ON AEDs

Alcohol elimination is zero-order (nonlinear) when blood levels are high but becomes first-order as the level falls. Alcohol is metabolized into acetaldehyde by 2 enzyme systems: alcohol dehydrogenase (the major pathway, which is noninducible) and the microsomal ethanol oxidizing system. Acetaldehyde is metabolized to acetate by aldehyde dehydrogenase. Nearly half of Asians slowly metabolize acetaldehyde, causing alcohol intolerance.

The hepatic mixed-function oxygenase system metabolizes alcohol and some AEDs by converting lipophilic compounds into hydrophilic compounds. The system uses hydroxylation, demethylation, and glucuronidation. Acutely, alcohol inhibits AED metabolism by this system, but the effect has little clinical significance. Following chronic consumption of alcohol, enzyme induction leads to more rapid metabolism of AEDs such as phenytoin, phenobarbital, and carbamazepine. Thus, individuals who chronically and excessively consume alcohol may require higher doses and more frequent dosing of these AEDs.

MARIJUANA

Marijuana, *Cannabis sativa*, is obtained from the flowering tops of hemp plants. Used medically for thousands of years, its popularity grew among 19th-century European physicians for various disorders, including epilepsy (2). Because of side effects, abuse, and introduction of synthetic medications, the Marijuana Tax Act of 1937 removed it from U.S. formularies (2–3). Its illicit but popular use never waned, and medical interest in marijuana and cannabidiols has increased significantly in the past several decades. Disorders for which cannabinoids have been postulated to be beneficial include emesis, pain, inflammation, anorexia, multiple sclerosis, neurodegenerative disorders (Parkinson disease, Huntington disease, Alzheimer disease), Tourette syndrome, epilepsy, glaucoma, osteoporosis, schizophrenia, cardiovascular disorders, cancer, obesity, and metabolic syndrome–related disorders (4). However, evidence that the benefits clearly outweigh the risks for long-term use are lacking in almost all disorders.

The main psychoactive agent in marijuana is tetrahydrocannabinol (THC), but most marijuana leaves contain numerous cannabidiols. These compounds can have complex and differing effects on seizure threshold and other neural actions. These compounds work mainly through their effects on the cannabidiol receptors in the brain (5). The 2 cannabidiol receptors (CB1 and CB2) where THC and other cannabidiols bind are G-coupled protein receptors. Endogenous cannabinoids appear to break synaptic circuits and regulate diverse physiologic and pathologic states, including neuronal excitability, regulation of food intake, immunomodulation, inflammation, pain, addictive behavior, and cancer (6). The CB1 receptor is found on presynaptic terminals, where it modulates calcium or potassium conductance, usually decreasing neuronal excitability and neurotransmitter release (7–8).

The anticonvulsant effects are postulated to occur at CB1 receptors via inhibition of glutamate release. Cannabidiols may have proconvulsant effects by activating or altering release of inhibitory neurotransmitters such as γ-aminobutyric acid (9). Animal studies suggest that THC and cannabidiols can have both antiepileptic as well as seizure-provoking effects.

The biological effects of marijuana on seizure threshold are complex, varying by chemical composition of the plant variety, epilepsy models, dosages, duration of therapy, and species (10). Anticonvulsant and antikindling properties predominate in most animal models for THC and cannabidiol (9–12). However, if THC and cannabidiol increase seizure threshold, then withdrawal of these compounds might provoke seizure activity. Animal studies demonstrate a withdrawal effect to THC (13). Thus, marijuana use could potentially provoke withdrawal seizures in some patients.

Human studies of marijuana for epilepsy are limited by small sample size, lack of adequate controls, and study duration. Short-term studies are mixed: 2 show efficacy, while one does not (14–16). A study of illicit drug use and risk of new-onset seizures showed that marijuana was associated with a decreased first seizure in men (17). Anecdotal cases suggest that marijuana can reduce seizure frequency in some patients but cause seizures in others (10, 18). The limits of anecdotal cases are legend.

Marijuana use is common in people with epilepsy. Among a consecutive series of patients readmitted to a South African hospital, 24% abused cannabis (19). Among 98 people with epilepsy who responded to a survey in New Mexico, nearly a third of those younger than 30 years used marijuana; most reported no effect on seizures (20). In a Canadian survey of 136 adult people with epilepsy, 21% actively used marijuana. None felt that marijuana exacerbated seizures; 68% reported improved seizure severity, and 54% reported reduced seizure frequency. However, there was a trend for active users to have higher seizure frequency and a longer duration of epilepsy than other groups (21).

The relative benefits and toxicity of marijuana, THC, and cannabidiol remain poorly defined in people with epilepsy. Since marijuana is illegal in most states and side effects occur, marijuana is not recommended to treat epilepsy. Further, as with alcohol, even if marijuana or one of its components had antiepileptic effects, abrupt withdrawal of moderate to high consumption should be avoided. Controlled trials are needed.

COCAINE

Cocaine can cause seizures and fatal arrhythmias. All forms of cocaine consumption can cause seizures within seconds to hours. Seizures caused by cocaine are uniquely dangerous and may be associated with myocardial ischemia, cardiac arrhythmias, and death. Cocaine-induced seizures can occur in someone who has never had a seizure. Cocaine should never be consumed by a person with known or suspected epilepsy.

AMPHETAMINES

Amphetamines, like cocaine, are stimulants. They are prescribed to treat attention deficit/hyperactivity disorder and narcolepsy. When used under a physician's supervision, amphetamines and other stimulants are safe for most children and adults with epilepsy. However, they can cause sleep deprivation, which is a common provocative factor for seizures. Abuse of amphetamines and other stimulants (e.g., crystal meth) can cause severe sleep deprivation, confusion, psychosis, and seizures. Overdoses of amphetamines can cause severe tonic-clonic seizures, heart attacks, and death.

Caffeine, present in coffee, tea, chocolate, and other foods, is the most commonly used psychoactive drug in the world. Caffeine is a bitter, white, crystalline alkaloid and is a natural pesticide that protects plants from insects. Its main action is as a nonselective antagonist of adenosine receptors; it also inhibits phosphodiesterase. Caffeine is a stimulant. The caffeine content of a cup of various beverages varies widely: green tea (30 mg), black tea (50 mg), coffee (80–125 mg in regular and 10 mg in decaffeinated), and Coca-Cola (35 mg). Caffeine is rapidly absorbed (within 45 minutes) and undergoes first-order kinetics with a half-life of approximately 5 hours. There is no evidence that caffeine directly alters the seizure threshold in humans. However, a related methylxanthine and metabolite of caffeine is theophylline. Theophylline is used to treat asthma, and it lowers the seizure threshold. However, since only 4% of coffee is metabolized to theophylline, this does not appear to be clinically relevant. Although caffeine does not cause seizures directly, since it is a stimulant and can cause insomnia, a secondary effect of caffeine could be sleep deprivation and a lower seizure threshold.

NICOTINE

Nicotine is an alkaloid most commonly obtained from tobacco; however, it is found in a variety of plants in the nightshade family. Nicotine is a stimulant and leads to dependence with long-term use. It is absorbed readily after inhalation, reaching the brain within 15 seconds. Its half-life is approximately 2 hours. The main physiologic effects are stimulation of nicotinic acetylcholine receptors in both the peripheral and central nervous systems. Nicotine is not known to have clinically significant effects on seizure threshold, except perhaps to increase seizure threshold in autosomal dominant nocturnal frontal lobe epilepsy. Cigarette smoking also can be dangerous in persons who have seizures that impair consciousness or motor control since an unextinguished cigarette can cause a fire. Also, bupropion (Zyban, Wellbutrin) is effective in helping smokers to quit but can lower the seizure threshold.

REFERENCES

1. Jackson H. Evolution and dissolution of the nervous system. *Lancet*. 1884;1:555–558.
2. Robson P. Therapeutic aspects of cannabis and cannabinoids. *Br J Psychiatry*. 2001;178: 107–115.

 3. Sirven JI, Berg AT. Marijuana as a treatment for epilepsy and multiple sclerosis? A "grass roots" movement. *Neurology.* 2004;62:1924–1925.
 4. Kogan NM, Mechoulam R. Cannabinoids in health and disease. *Dialogues Clin Neurosci.* 2007;9:413–430.
 5. Pistis M, Melis M. From surface to nuclear receptors: the endocannabinoid family extends its assets. *Curr Med Chem.* 2010;17:1450–1467.
 6. Guindon J, Beaulieu P. The role of endogenous cannabinoid system in peripheral analgesia. *Curr Mol Pharmacol.* 2009;2:134–139.
 7. Guindon J, Hohmann AG. The endocannabinoid system and pain. *CNS Neurol Disord Drug Targets.* 2009;8:403–421.
 8. Elphick MR, Egertova M. The neurobiology and evolution of cannabinoid signaling. *Philos Trans R Soc Lond B Biol Sci.* 2001;356:381–408.
 9. Smith PF. Cannabinoids as potential anti-epileptic drugs. *Curr Opin Investig Drugs.* 2005;6:680–685.
10. Mortati K, Dworetzky B, Devinsky O. Marijuana: an effective antiepileptic treatment in partial epilepsy? A case report and review of the literature. *Rev Neurol Dis.* 2007;4: 103–106.
11. Wada JA, Osawa T, Corcoran ME. Effects of tetrahydrocannabinols on kindled amygdaloid seizures and photogenic seizures in Senegalese baboons, *Papio papio. Epilepsia.* 1975;16: 439–448.
12. Chiu P, Olsen DM, Borys HK, Karler R, Turkanis SA. The influence of cannabidiol and delta-9-tetrahydrocannabinol on cobalt epilepsy in rats. *Epilepsia.* 1979;20:365–375.
13. Karler R, Turkanis SA. The cannabinoids as potential antiepileptics. *J Clin Pharmacol.* 1981;21:S437–S448.
14. Cunha JM, Carlini EA, Pereira AE, et al. Chronic administration of cannabidiol to healthy volunteers and epileptic patients. *Pharmacology.* 1980;21:175–185.
15. Drysdale AJ, Platt B. Cannabinoids: mechanisms and therapeutic applications in the CNS. *Curr Med Chem.* 2003;10:2719–2732.
16. Ames FR, Cridland S. Anticonvulsant effect of cannabidiol. *S Afr Med J.* 1986;69:14.
17. Ng SK, Brust JC, Hauser WA, Susser M. Illicit drug use and the risk of new-onset seizures. *Am J Epidemiol.* 1990;132:47–57.
18. Keeler MH, Reifler CB. Grand mal convulsions subsequent to marijuana use. *Dis Nerv Syst.* 1967;28:474–475.
19. Saha SK, Nel M, Prinsloo EA. Profile and associated factors for re-admitted epileptic patients with complications in a South African hospital. *Cent Afr J Med.* 2006;52:35–38.
20. Feeney DM. Letter: marihuana use among epileptics. *JAMA.* 1976;235:1105.
21. Gross DW, Hamm J, Ashworth NL, Quigley D. Marijuana use and epilepsy: prevalence in patients of a tertiary care epilepsy center. *Neurology.* 2004;62:2095–2097.

16

Environmental Factors and Epilepsy

When seizures occur unexpectedly in people with epilepsy (PWE), careful investigation often uncovers recurrent triggers. After medication-related factors, hormonal influences, and intrinsic causes of enhanced epileptogenicity are excluded, a search for external provocative factors may be revealing. Common behavioral precipitants, such as sleep deprivation and extraordinary emotional stress, as well as withdrawal from excessive alcohol intake are well-known causes of unexpected seizures and are discussed in detail throughout this book. Environmental changes, on the other hand, while more difficult to implicate, play a role in some breakthrough seizures. Excessive heat or cold, intense sensory stimulation, sudden startle, and high altitudes may stress the body and lower seizure thresholds. In some cases, the environmental stimuli are very specific, such as a certain type of music or a certain mental activity (e.g., chess). For each PWE, potential environmental stressors should be identified and minimized, or seizures may persist despite appropriate medical management.

WEATHER

People with epilepsy sometimes complain of seizures during abrupt climate change. In patient surveys, weather is cited as a frequent seizure trigger (1). While controlled studies of climate effects on epilepsy do not exist, animal models demonstrate seasonal variations in antiepileptic drug (AED) efficacy (2–3). For PWE, it is possible that rapidly rising or falling temperatures may cause seizures by affecting neuronal function directly or indirectly through metabolic, vascular, or hormonal alterations. Dehydration from excessive heat or hypothermia from intense cold result in intense metabolic stress, and seizure threshold is likely to be reduced. More subtle effects of temperature change on seizure control may play a role in susceptible patients but are harder to implicate and even harder to avoid. Other possible seasonal changes in epilepsy include increased infantile spasms in winter and a higher winter birth rate for PWE.

Temperature may not be the only important weather effect on seizures. In a study of seizure occurrence in an epilepsy monitoring unit, large changes in atmospheric pressure (AP) were associated with increased seizure risk (4). The authors speculate about possible causes, including the direct effect of high and low barometric pressures as well as the change in the partial pressure of oxygen that occurs with AP change. Additional studies are needed to confirm these findings.

The role of sunlight exposure and risk for epilepsy and seizures remains unclear. One UK researcher has proposed that sunlight exposure and phototherapy may reduce the risk of seizures (5). Support for the hypothesis includes epidemiologic studies reporting higher prevalence rates for epilepsy in northern compared to southern European countries, animal models, and a complex role for melatonin and vitamin D in PWE. The association remains controversial, and definitive studies are lacking.

LUNAR PHASES

Throughout history, the full moon has been blamed for numerous medical and psychological (i.e., lunacy) ailments, but scientific evidence is lacking for most associations. In 2001, a large retrospective study of 3,757 patients who had breast surgery concluded that lunar phase had no effect on surgical survival rates (6). On the other hand, a recent study of admissions to an Austrian stroke unit revealed a statistically significant increase in admissions for nonmedical causes of strokelike symptoms during the full moon (7).

The largest study of the effect of lunar phase in epilepsy was performed as a 5-year retrospective review of seizure admissions to a Greek emergency department (8). Seizure admissions for both men and women increased by approximately 12% during full-moon days compared with other phases, which is a statistically significant finding. If the study conclusions are correct and reproducible, the cause is unclear. Speculation about gravitational effects, electromagnetic field changes, and sleep deprivation from enhanced ambient lighting were considered possible causes.

ALTITUDE AND SEIZURES

At high altitude, the brain is exposed to low AP combined with low partial pressures of oxygen. Adverse consequences range from headache to acute mountain sickness to frank cerebral edema (9). The severity of illness often correlates with the rapidity of ascent to altitudes above 3,000 m without time for the body to adapt to the relative hypoxia (10). In severe cases, massive cerebral edema, hypoxia, and cerebral hypoperfusion cause seizures from brain injury. Fortunately, cases of severe cerebral edema are rare. However, the risk of milder forms of

Table 16.1 High Altitude and Recommendations for People with Epilepsy

1. Staged ascent
2. Avoid tobacco, alcohol, sleeping pills, and narcotics
3. Avoid strenuous activity for the first 24 h after arrival to each new altitude
4. Limit gains of elevation to 300 m/d, and for every 1000 m, spend a day to acclimatize
5. Climb high, sleep low
6. Good hydration: as much as 3 to 4 qt of free water a day
7. Prophylactic medications for a history of a spectrum of high-altitude illnesses

Reproduced with permission from Maa (11).

altitude sickness or even subclinical effects on seizure threshold for the PWE is more likely and difficult to quantify. From 2001 to 2005, 27 of an estimated 2 million visitors per year to Colorado's Summit County were treated for generalized seizures (11). All patients lived at altitudes below 2,000 m and had seizures within an average of 2.5 days from arrival. Nearly half were first-time seizures, and the rest occurred in patients with prior seizure history. As none of the patients exhibited signs of pulmonary or cerebral edema, the exact contribution of altitude change is unknown. However, sleep disturbances and headaches were frequently reported prior to seizures, suggesting a physiologic effect of higher altitudes. Proposed altitude-related, pathophysiologic mechanisms include mild cerebral edema, sleep deprivation, hyperventilation, and the direct effects of hypobaric hypoxia (11) (Table 16.1).

For PWE with a history of seizures related to altitude, possible preventive measures include assuring therapeutic levels of existing AEDs, increasing maintenance doses of AEDs, and supplementation with acetazolamide (12). Acetazolamide is a carbonic anhydrase inhibitor that may help drive ventilation by lowering the serum pH, resulting in less hypoxia. Additionally, by reducing production of cerebrospinal fluid, acetazolamide may help prevent cerebral edema. The usual adult dose is 125 to 250 mg twice daily for adults initiated 1 or 2 days before climbing and continuing for 2 to 3 days after the highest elevation is reached.

VISUAL STIMULI: FLASHING LIGHTS, BRIGHT LIGHTS AND TELEVISIONS, AND VIDEO GAMES

In electroencephalographic (EEG) studies, up to 3% of people exposed to flashing lights or patterns are photosensitive and exhibit focal or generalized EEG abnormalities (13). Photosensitivity is more common in children and females (14). Far fewer people, approximately 1 in 10,000, have seizures induced by visual stimuli. When seizures occur, generalized tonic-clonic, myoclonic, and absence seizures are the most likely types (15). In PWE, the incidence of photosensitivity varies tremendously with epilepsy subtype. For the relatively rare disorders, including the progressive myoclonic epilepsies and Dravet syndrome, photosensitive seizures affect nearly half of all individuals. Among the more prevalent epilepsies, light- and pattern-induced seizures are most common in the generalized or idiopathic epilepsy syndromes. Photosensitivity is less likely in the acquired partial or localization-related seizure disorders, and when it does occur, EEGs usually reveal more restricted abnormalities and therefore a reduced threat of seizures compared with generalized syndromes (14).

While high-intensity strobe lights like those used during EEG may precipitate seizures, they are uncommonly encountered outside of nightclubs and theaters. More ubiquitous stimuli include flickering or flashing lights emanating from faulty fluorescent lighting, light filtering through trees along a road, light reflected off water, and flashing patterns on televisions and computer screens. Seizures are more likely when visual stimulation is bright, of high contrast, and at frequencies of 15 to 25 Hz (13). Some studies suggest red flickering light is more provocative than other colors. In addition to intense flashing lights, viewing patterns may induce seizures. Parallel lines and stripes, either stationary or oscillating, seem to induce the most seizures compared with other shapes and patterns (16–17). Table 16.2 lists recommendations for reducing the risk of seizures from visual stimulation.

Watching television may induce seizures in photosensitive individuals. The flicker caused by the scan rate of a television may be experienced when sitting very close to the screen. Because of the scan rates, European televisions (which may result in a flicker of 50 Hz) may induce seizures more readily than American televisions (may flicker at 60 Hz) (18). The risk may be reduced by increasing distance from the screen and/or by adding ambient light. It is likely that newer LCD and LED flat screen televisions and computer screens with much faster refresh rates may reduce the risk. However, the broadcast content is important. A 1997 broadcast of a Pokemon cartoon in Japan containing a rocket launch sequence with flashing red and blue light resulted in over 500 children having seizures, most of whom had no history of seizure disorder. Since that time, program screening methods and recommendations for limiting flickering

Table 16.2 Precautions for Photosensitive Patients

View television from ≥8 ft

View television in a well-lit room with a small lamp on top of the TV set

Do not approach the TV set to adjust or switch channels

Cover one eye if it is necessary to go near the TV

Avoid discotheques or places with flashing lights

Wear polarized glasses on sunny days to reduce flickering reflections from water, etc.

Adapted from Harding and Jeavons (17).

stimuli have been developed to limit exposure to provocative content in television programs.

Video and computer games can also cause seizures in photosensitive patients. For PWE with a history of seizures provoked by video game play or those with photosensitivity on EEG and seizures provoked by video game play, it is likely that the games are a trigger for seizures and represent a real risk. As a result, video game industry guidelines in the United Kingdom and Japan recommend limiting bright flashes at frequencies higher than 3 per second and ensuring that light-dark stationary, oscillating, or reversing patterns have more than 5 stripes unless they are restricted to less than 25% of the screen or are less than 50 cd/m^2 in brightness (13). Patients with partial (localization-related) epilepsy without photosensitive EEG abnormalities are much less likely to have seizures triggered by video games (19). However, seizures still may occur as an indirect consequence, possibly the result of excitement, intense concentration, or fatigue.

TRAVEL

People with epilepsy may be vulnerable to breakthrough seizures when traveling. Traveling is stressful, especially by air. Security lines, delayed flights, lost luggage, new surroundings and the unexpected all cause stress. Additionally, night flights and time zone changes alter medication schedules and cause jet lag and sleep deprivation, lowering seizure thresholds. A small 2006 study analyzed the effect of air travel on seizure frequency in 37 PWE (20). While the patients had no in-flight events, seizures were statistically more likely to occur the week after flying. Poorly controlled seizures at baseline, history of seizures after travel, and excessive worry about seizures during flights predicted travel-related seizures.

Physicians caring for PWE should review travel plans carefully with their patients. In some cases, increasing maintenance doses and AED serum levels prior to travel is appropriate. Ensuring sleep on night flights and premedication of anxious patients with low-dose benzodiazepines may be reasonable, especially when a history of travel-related seizures exists.

REFERENCES

1. Spatt J, Langbauer G, Mamoli B. Subjective perception of seizure precipitants: results of a questionnaire study. *Seizure*. 1998;7:391–395.
2. Torshin VI, Vlasova IG. Biorhythmologic aspects of seizure activity. *Bull Exp Biol Med*. 2001;132:1025–1028.
3. Loscher W, Fiedler M. The role of technical, biological, and pharmacological factors in the laboratory evaluation of anticonvulsant drugs. VII. Seasonal influences on anticonvulsant drug actions in mouse models of generalized seizures. *Epilepsy Res*. 2000;38:231–248.
4. Doherty MJ, Youn C, Gwinn RP, Haltiner AM. Atmospheric pressure and seizure frequency in the epilepsy unit: preliminary observations. *Epilepsia*. 2007;48:1674–1767.
5. Baxendale SA. Light therapy as a treatment for epilepsy. *Med Hypotheses*. 2011;76: 661–664.

6. Peters-Engl C, Frank W, Kerschbaum F, Denison U, Medl M, Sevelda P. Lunar phases and survival of breast cancer patients—a statistical analysis of 3,757 cases. *Breast Cancer Res Treat*. 2001;70:131–135.

7. Baumgartner RW, Siegel AM, Hackett PH. Going high with preexisting neurological conditions. *High Alt Med Biol*. 2007;8:108–116.

8. Polychronopoulos P, Argyriou AA, Sirrou V. Lunar phases and seizure occurrence: just an ancient legend? *Neurology*. 2006;66:1442–1443.

9. Wilson MH, Newman S, Imray CH. The cerebral effects of ascent to high altitudes. *Lancet Neurol*. 2009;8:175–191.

10. Imray C, Wright A, Subudhi A, Roach R. Acute mountain sickness: pathophysiology, prevention, and treatment. *Prog Cardiovasc Dis*. 2010;52:467–484.

11. Maa EH. How do you approach seizures in the high altitude traveler? *High Alt Med Biol*. 2011;12:13–19.

12. Maa EH. Hypobaric hypoxic cerebral insults: the neurological consequences of going higher. *NeuroRehabilitation*. 2010;26:73–84.

13. Fisher RS, Harding G, Erba G, Barkley GL, Wilkins A, Epilepsy Foundation of America Working Group. Photic- and pattern-induced seizures: a review for the Epilepsy Foundation of America Working Group. *Epilepsia*. 2005;46:1426–1441.

14. Lu Y, Waltz S, Stenzel K, Muhle H, Stephani U. Photosensitivity in epileptic syndromes of childhood and adolescence. *Epileptic Disord*. 2008;10:136–143.

15. Covanis A. Photosensitivity in idiopathic generalized epilepsies. *Epilepsia*. 2005;46:67–72.

16. Jeavons PM, Harding GF. Photosensitive epilepsy: a review of the literature and a study of 460 patients. In: *Clinics in Developmental Medicine*. No. 56. London, England: William Heineman Medical Books; 1975:1–121.

17. Harding GFA. Jeavons PM. *Photosensitive Epilepsy*. London, England: MacKeith Press; 1994.

18. Tassinari CA, Rubboli G, Rizzi R, Gardella E, Michelucci R. Self-induction of visually-induced seizures. *Adv Neurol*. 1998;75:179–192.

19. Millett CJ, Fish DR, Thompson PJ, et al. Seizures during videogame play and other common leisure pursuits in known epilepsy patients without visual sensitivity. *Epilepsia* 1999:40(suppl 4):59–64.

20. Trevorrow T. Air travel and seizure frequency for individuals with epilepsy. *Seizure*. 2006;15:320–327.

Appendix

LEVELS OF EVIDENCE IN MEDICAL SCIENCE

Physicians decide about treating patients based on many kinds of information, including published reports of well-controlled clinical trials, case series and individual case reports, expert opinion, and personal experience. Evidence-based medicine is a discipline that seeks to use the most scientifically accurate information to make medical decisions. The data used to assess the risks and benefits of a diagnostic study or treatment can be divided into many levels, but an overview is presented in the Table.

Randomized, Controlled Clinical Trials

Randomization in a clinical trial is the chance assignment of a patient to active treatment or to a non-treatment control group. The control group receives a placebo, which is an inactive substance. In an active placebo study, one group receives a very low dose of medication or electrical stimulation from a device that is considered subtherapeutic and the other group receives a higher dose. The patients in the two treatment groups have similar traits, such as the extent of disease. Only authorized researchers may administer the study, which is typically sponsored by the National Institutes of Health, a pharmaceutical company, or a private institution.

The trial follows a detailed protocol that includes the study goals, inclusion and exclusion criteria, number of patients in treatment and placebo groups, evaluation tools, and primary and secondary outcome measures.

In a blinded study, the patient does not know whether the medication or stimulation they receive is the active or placebo agent. In a double-blind study, neither the patients nor the investigators know who receives the medication/ stimulation and who receives the inactive therapy. Blinding eliminates biases such as the expectation of improvement or adverse effects.

211

Evidence-Based Data

Evidentiary Level	Study Type	Notes
I	At least one well-designed randomized controlled trial	Statistical significance does not equal clinical significance. Large, well-powered studies often show statistical effects but do not provide meaningful benefits.
II	Well-designed controlled trials that were not randomized	Lack of randomization can lead to selection bias. For example, patients who volunteer for a study may have greater disease severity and be less likely to benefit from therapy, thereby negatively biasing a study.
III	Well-designed cohort or case-control analytic studies, usually from more than one research group.	These clinical or epidemiological studies often look at a broad population at a moment in time rather than prospectively over time. Many issues can complicate the interpretation of these studies, such as sample bias and the danger of mistaking an association for a cause-effect relationship.
IV	Multiple uncontrolled case series or dramatic results in uncontrolled trials	Results may be due to chance or from unknown factors. Often subject to bias of patient and investigator. Also potential bias of funding source (e.g., pharmaceutical/device company).
V	Case studies	Most valuable as suggesting a possible insight into mechanism of disease or effectiveness of an intervention. Large potential to attribute a causal relation to something that is really due to chance, placebo effect, or other factors.

Observational Studies

Investigators can study the causes and treatments by using observational studies – careful observations, such as practice audits, based on the results of various treatments. These are *neither controlled nor randomized* studies. In some cases, it may be unethical to randomize patients. For example, if one wanted to study the effect of parental love on seizure control in children ages 3 to 5 years, it would be unethical to randomize half of a group of children to "minimal love" where parents left children alone for longer times and displayed less physical affection. In other studies, it may be too costly or too difficult to randomize patients prospectively. For example, it would be unrealistic to randomize half of an epilepsy population to a 20 gram per day carbohydrate vs. unrestricted diet but have no resources for dietary counseling about what foods are allowed nor efforts to assess compliance.

The lack of control and randomization allows the potential for selection bias. Thus, if one compares patients in one group versus those in another, their difference may not reflect the variable you are interested in (e.g., a medical or alternative therapy), but some other factor that led them to seek that therapy or lifestyle. For example, obese individuals may have changes in their hormonal milieu that change their selection of diet. So diet may influence weight, but weight may influence diet as well. In epilepsy, an example is the efficacy of seizure alert dogs. Some very positive responses occurred in patients with seizures due to conversion disorder but not epilepsy. It suggests that patients with conversion may be more prone to seek certain therapeutic interventions and to report positive outcomes. The positive responses may not reflect the intervention but the group of patients who chose to receive the intervention.

Epidemiological research studies the incidence, distribution, and control of illness in populations, and how various influences (diet, lifestyle, environment, medication) cause, prevent, or improve the disease.

Case Studies

Case studies include published case reports as well as cases that are compiled informally, or orally shared with colleagues. Studying one patient at a time offers advantages of intimate knowledge and an ability to enmesh oneself in the personal, social as well as medical aspects of a life. Clinical details focus on the potential causes, symptoms, treatment, and outcome of a specific patient's illness. The patient interview, often supplemented by family and other witnesses, provides important statements about medical history, symptoms, responses to treatment, and quality of life, the patient's ability to enjoy life. Lessons from individual patients abound, but there are many dangers. Case studies can suggest a clear causal relationship when the association is due to coincidence, the placebo effect, or may be a non-causal but significantly associated factor. For example, an adolescent may take a new vitamin tablet and for the first time in months not have a seizure during sleep. A month later, the vitamin is taken again and once again the patient is seizure free that night after having seizures every other night. Coincidence is unlikely. This case strongly suggests that the vitamin controls the seizure as no other medicines were changed. However, the real variable was sleeping over at grandmother's home, where she received the vitamin. There, instead of sharing a room with two noisy and annoying siblings, she slept alone and fully. Improved seizure control was from better sleep, not the vitamin.

Index